Vital Sensation Manual

UNIT FIVE:
VITAL EXPRESSION
A MANUAL ON HOMEOPATHIC
CASETAKING

Based on
The Sensation Method
& Classical Homeopathy

Written
by
Melissa Burch, CCH, RsHom(NA) & Didi Pershouse, CCH

Cover Design by Chetana Deorah

Layout and Design by Janet Innes

Edited by Debi Levine

Published by
Inner Health, Inc.
175 Harvey St., #13
Cambridge, MA 02140
(617) 491-3374
melissa@innerhealth.us
www.innerhealth.us

© 2011, Inner Health, Inc.

I would like to express my gratitude to Dr. Jayesh Shah and Julian Jonas, whose teaching and encouragement have been the foundation of my successful practice.
— Didi Pershouse, 2007

Dr. Rajan Sankaran's masterful approach to homeopathy and his breakthrough to understand "sensation" and "source" in our cases has revolutionized homeopathy. I am forever grateful for his teachings and ideas that have inspired this manual.

— Melissa Burch, 2007

TABLE OF CONTENTS

INTRODUCTION

We are at an exciting age in homeopathy. A new science of systems-based homeopathy is developing that will allow both wider and more accurate prescribing. Homeopaths from widely diverging philosophies are beginning to see patterns emerging that link families of remedies with patterns in the body and mind. The advent, in the past decade, of computer search engines within homeopathic databases has allowed homeopaths to see these larger groupings of information—by analyzing the common language, symptoms and sensations expressed in cured cases and provings within families of related remedies.

By applying these findings, and working with the actual language and gestures of the patient, a new way of taking the case has been developed that allows the homeopath to reliably determine the Kingdom (plant, animal, mineral, etc.) of the remedy the patient needs, as well as the Sub-kingdom, and the Source itself.

The Sensation Method is not theoretical; it comes directly from the patient, who can—with gentle guidance—usually go from a full exploration of his main complaint to an accurate description of the qualities of the remedy he needs. This can only happen, however, if the practitioner's questions follow a certain logical order. In the past few years there has been much confusion over the proper application of this seemingly magical game of getting the patient to describe or even name the remedy needed. There have been many homeopaths who, with the best intentions, abandoned all their previous knowledge to chase after an endless stream of images given by their patients, with disastrous results. This has led to onlookers shaking their heads in dismay--since it appears that if the patient mentions a lion, the homeopath immediately prescribes Lac Leoninum. Because of this unfortunate misuse of this process, some homeopaths dismiss the Sensation Method as pure fancy.

Still other homeopaths have a solid understanding of what they are looking for with this method, but apply a disorganized casetaking style. Many homeopaths successfully use the "follow the energy" approach. This works well for homeopaths experienced with the Sensation Method, and particularly intuitive types. But for homeopaths new to the Sensation Method, there is a lot of confusion about what "following the energy" means and how to understand what "energy" to follow in the case. The Vital Expression approach to casetaking helps to alleviate many common mistakes by giving a sequence of steps the homeopath can use when taking and/or analyzing the case.

The Sensation Method, though often referred to as the "New" Method, is soundly based on the foundations of classical homeopathy and the Organon, including the principles of "like cures like," minimum dosages, single remedies, the concept of miasms, finding the strange, rare and peculiar, and even

Hahnemann's own warnings about the potential misuse of the Doctrine of Signatures.

This manual outlines a step-by-step method to find the remedy using the Sensation Method by identifying the Vital Expression. We do not intend to say that this is the only way to find the Source or follow the Vital Expression. Nor do we expect this to be the final word. Homeopathic casetaking and analysis is changing rapidly, and many people are contributing new and wonderful ideas, all of which will have to be tried, tested, and integrated over time. This manual is simply an outline of one way that we have found to be reliable, effective, and easily applicable for most people.

GOALS OF THIS MANUAL

We expect this manual to help you to:

- Know where you are in the case.
- Know what information is still required.
- Recognize which level the patient is speaking from.
- Know what kinds of questions to ask at each point during the casetaking.
- Recognize the Vital Expression, (formerly called Vital Sensation).
- Know the difference between Miasm language and Vital Expression language.
- Know when you are hearing Kingdom and Sub-kingdom language.*
- Know when the patient is giving you a description of the Source.
- Know when you have enough information and are ready to prescribe a remedy.
- Recognize when the case is not clear, and other methods should be used to determine the best remedy.

Note: The full, in-depth process of analyzing the Sub-kingdom is beyond the scope of this manual, though we have introduced it up to a point. Fortunately the research and publishing of Materia Medica organized by Sub-kingdoms is continuously growing through the work of many homeopaths and is the basis of improving homeopathy for all.

PART 1: THE SENSATION METHOD

The Sensation Method versus Other Methods

Different ways of analyzing cases have evolved throughout the history of homeopathy, all of which are still being used today. The most common ways are listed below:

- Keynote Prescribing
- Mental and Emotional Characteristics
- Common Personality Pictures of Remedies
- Delusional and Thematic prescribing

    And now…
- The Sensation Method (sometimes called The New Method or the Bombay Group Method)

Hazards of the Other Methods

Many patients throughout the world have been helped using a variety of methods, and all these methods have contributed to our understanding of homeopathy. Why do we need another method? The other methods each have something to offer, but they also have shortcomings. Common problems with other methods of practice include the following:

- **Homeopath centered.** What needs to be cured is often determined by the homeopath, not the patient.

- **Abandoning the Chief Complaint.** The Chief Complaint is often abandoned in order to explore areas that the homeopath deems more important, leaving patients to feel they are being psychoanalyzed, rather than being treated for their actual complaints.

- **Seeing only certain parts of the case.** Remedies are often chosen based on a few keynotes, without reflecting the entire picture being presented by the patient.

- **Unclear prescribing.** Kingdoms and miasms are often unclear and not used in finding the prescription; therefore, the chance of finding the correct remedy is diminished.

- **Theorizing.** The other methods use a lot of theorizing and interpreting about where the center of the case is, rather than taking information directly from the patient.

What Distinguishes the Sensation Method?

- **Patient Centered.** The *patient* is the one who determines the topic of most importance and the Chief Complaint. The homeopath trusts that the patient is the most accurate judge of what needs to be cured.

- **Based on the Chief Complaint.** The Sensation Method explores the Chief Complaint completely. The story and emotions are explored only to the extent that they flow out of the discussion of the Chief Complaint; therefore, the patient and homeopath can see their relevance.

- **Deeper understanding.** The Sensation Method seeks the deepest level of the patient's individual experience or Vital Expression, and through this Vital Expression understands the Kingdom, Sub-kingdom and Source material of the remedy that is needed.

- **More accurate prescribing.** In many cases taken with the Sensation Method, the homeopath can get information directly from the patient about the Source of the remedy he or she needs. This is of particular benefit when a patient needs an unusual or unknown remedy which the homeopath would never find by repertorizing. The description of the substance is more reliable than the naming of the Source.

- **Less interpretation.** The Sensation Method lessens the chance of any rational, emotional or cultural interpretation in analyzing a case. Instead, the homeopath learns to "Pattern Match" the patient's Universal or non-human-specific Language to a specific Kingdom, Sub-kingdom and Source.

Pitfalls of the Sensation Method When Not Used Properly

The Sensation Method has many benefits. However, it is only effective if used properly. If you do not have a firm grasp of the concepts of the Sensation Method, your prescriptions will be inaccurate. It is better to stick with the other methods than to be confused or make assumptions in your cases—especially when your prescription is not based on traditional homeopathic principles. Here are some of the most common pitfalls of using the Sensation Method without fully understanding it.

Expecting patients to name a substance. Now that we know it is possible, everyone wants their patient to name the substance they need. But in actuality, most of the time that people are speaking at Source level, they cannot access the name of what they are describing. They can only give the qualities. If you prescribe based on the substances they name without understanding the qualities of the Source, most likely you are not prescribing the Source remedy.

Prescribing based on an image. In the Sensation Method there has been a lot of confusion between Delusional/Image language and Source language. Without understanding the map of proper casetaking, it can be easy to prescribe on an image based on Delusional language, which is useless, unless you happen to get lucky. But luck is not replicable or reliable.

Throwing out your foundation of knowledge. There has been a tendency for people to throw out previous knowledge, including repertorization and use of the Materia Medica, in their rush to use the Sensation Method. This is a very bad idea because the basic principles of homeopathy are confirmed in this Method.

Sloppy initial casetaking leading to numerous recases. The experience of exploring the Vital Expression and going to Source can be intense for some patients. In tough cases, the patient may be reluctant to go through the extensive questioning more than once, so you want to find the best remedy on the initial casetaking.

Looking for a single sensation, as opposed to a whole pattern. There has been a misunderstanding that the "Vital Sensation" (Vital Expression) is a single thing or word that the homeopath is looking for. In most cases, however, it turns out to be a complex pattern encompassing many sensations. This misunderstanding has led many people to prescribe based on a single word or two. For example, they think 'pressure' plus 'hard' must indicate a Mineral case.

Leaving out what doesn't fit. When you get an idea for a remedy too early on, the patient may say numerous expressions that do not fit in the way you understand the case—so you just ignore them. In many cases, however, these unusual statements are key to understanding the real prescription.

Only following what you already know. Sometimes, the homeopath forgets to look for the strange, rare and peculiar, and picks up something familiar to them but not really peculiar to the patient. And they push it and push it and push it. They end up seeing only what they want to see, without understanding the patient's actual experience. Then the information from the case is either incomplete, totally confusing, or misleading.

Confusing local sensations for Vital Expressions. If the local sensation that emerges from the Chief Complaint is not confirmed as the Vital Expression throughout the case, beginners using this method may assume that a local sensation is the Vital Expression. They then often jump to "Sankaran's Schema" and start looking up those sensation words in the Plant charts, or make an assumption about Kingdom too soon.

Relying on bypasses. Bypasses (such as asking about hobbies and favorite movies) have been taught as useful alternatives at certain points in the case, but in actuality, the prognosis is very poor when one has to use a bypass, so they should be used as little as possible. In children's cases, bypasses may be necessary to form a rapport, and there may be more energy in what the child wants to talk about than what the parent wants treated.

Working in isolation. We are early in the development of our ideas and cataloguing of cases by this method, and many homeopaths are trying to practice in a vacuum after a workshop or two on this method. Often a case does very well for a year or more, then the homeopath sees that the prescription needs refining. This often happens during an acute manifestation, when the patient can express the pattern more clearly. This is where working in groups that share cured cases and take the time to extract out the Kingdom, Sub-kingdom and Source language is an invaluable part of our development.

Lack of Confirmations. Homeopaths working in this method may mistakenly think they don't need to confirm their prescriptions. In all cases where the remedy is well-known, you must use traditional ways to confirm the prescription: i.e., the symptoms of the patient need to be checked in the Materia Medica and Repertory. If the remedy is well-proven and you do not find confirmatory rubrics, then you should seriously doubt your prescription. (If it is a lesser-known, unknown, or poorly-proven remedy and you don't find confirmatory rubrics, then your prescription *may* still be correct but your prognosis of cure reduces.)

How to Avoid the Pitfalls of the Sensation Method

If you follow the steps outlined in this manual, you can increase the reliability of your prescriptions and streamline your work, and avoid many of the pitfalls that homeopaths using the Sensation Method have experienced. The method outlined below is effective because it:

- Confirms the Kingdom at the "right" level.

- Produces more reliable Sub-kingdom information by reducing confusion between Fact level, Delusion level and Kingdom level.

- Elicits more reliable Source description language at the appropriate time during the case (when the patient is actually speaking from the level of Energy), rather than randomly collecting words to make a "picture."

- Streamlines the process of casetaking in an organized fashion.

- Reduces the need for retakes.

Myths and Truths about Using the Sensation Method

Myth: All your experience no longer applies.

Truth: All the time you have studied with other teachers is invaluable. If you lose that connection to your basic understanding of homeopathic theory, then your work will not be grounded in the foundations of homeopathic knowledge.

Myth: The Sensation Method disregards provings, rubrics, and the Materia Medica.

Truth: We don't use these as much to find the remedy. But we absolutely use all of it to *confirm* the remedy. If you find a well-known remedy and it is not matching what we already know about that remedy from the Materia Medica or provings, you should seriously doubt your prescription. However, if it's a very small remedy and there is not a lot of information from the original proving, then it's possible that what you see in this method may not be in the Materia Medica.

Myth: The Sensation Method isn't homeopathy at all. Hahnemann would be shocked.

Truth: In fact, the Sensation Method is firmly grounded in the basic principles outlined in the Organon. In some ways it is closer than much of what is practiced under the name of "Classical Homeopathy."

Myth: If you study the Sensation Method, you can't study any other method.

Truth: If you really understand this process, other workshops, teachers, and methods will add value, rather than being a distraction. Homeopathy is a continually expanding body of knowledge, and many teachers around the world are starting to see links between families of remedies and patterns in the body and mind. The Sensation Method is only one aspect of the emerging practice of systems-based homeopathy.

PART 2: SENSATION METHOD CONCEPTS

The Sensation Method uses concepts and terminology that may be unfamiliar to you. In this section, we will define those concepts and terms.

The Vital Expression (also called the Vital Sensation)

Dr. Rajan Sankaran has called the place where the body and mind express the same phenomena the "Vital Sensation," but we have found the term "Vital Expression" to be more useful (see below).

Dr. Sankaran wrote in "The Sensation in Homeopathy":

> "…the disease, the totality of the signs and symptoms, mental and physical, general and particular—all of this comes from our basic disturbance and that disturbance is not in the mind, nor in the body; it is something deeper than both. At that level the person talks a language which is both mental and physical. The body and the mind can then be seen as an expression of that level (sensation) and that language actually is not even the language of the human being. It is a language that comes from a Source that is different from the human being: a plant, a mineral or an animal."

The Vital Expression is the patient's experience of his or her state and its connection to the Vital Disturbance. Most patients are intimately familiar with the Vital Expression, but have never thought about it. But it is there all the time—like the heart beating. This Vital Expression is something you need the patient to articulate in order to fully understand the case. Homeopathy is language based, therefore the process of analysis and identifying the remedy proceeds directly from the language of the patient.

The Vital Expression can be brought into consciousness via the casetaking process, during which the patient will describe the Vital Expression using words, gestures, and images. They know exactly what they are talking about, but they may never have had a chance to describe it. They have been experiencing it their whole life, without ever being fully aware of it.

When you unlock this Vital Expression, the door opens and reveals the Kingdom, Sub-kingdom and Source. The Vital Expression is our connection to the universe. It has deep spiritual and philosophical resonance because it is a truth. Other traditions, such as Vipassana Meditation, have also described this phenomenon.

When chasing the Vital Expression, the client will travel through different levels of experiences, which represent his perspective of the world (from the superficial to the deepest core). The Vital Expression is repeated over and over in the case from the Chief Complaint, the other complaints, dreams, etc. This inner state of the patient can only be described using Universal Language (non-human specific language), which helps the homeopath to recognize the Kingdom, the Sub-kingdom and Source.

Every patient can go there. It is in them.

Why Change Vital Sensation' to 'Vital Expression?'

It is not *one* thing we are searching for in the case. The Vital Expression is a whole process that the patient intimately experiences, but may not be conscious of in their everyday life. We are changing "Vital Sensation" to "Vital Expression" because the term used needs to imply not *one* thing, but a whole process that is being shared through language and gesture.

Also, the Vital Expression is not a level itself, and is not found at only one level in the case. It manifests throughout the case, even in the fact, emotional and delusional levels. To call it 'Vital Sensation' creates confusion when distinguishing between "local sensations," "Sensation level" and what was previously called "Vital Sensation." So we have chosen to call it Vital Expression.

Kingdoms and Sub-kingdoms

The Sensation Method of Homeopathy is a systems-based method that looks for information about the Kingdom of the remedy that is needed by observing the patient's language and gestures at certain stages in the case. Kingdoms include: Plants, Animals, Minerals, Fungi, Nosodes, and Imponderables.

Sub-kingdoms are groupings within Kingdoms. In the Animal Kingdom, examples of Sub-kingdoms would be Mammals, Birds and Reptiles. In the Mineral Kingdom, remedies are grouped into Sub-kingdoms based on the Rows and Columns of the Periodic Table of Elements. Remedies from the Plant Kingdom are grouped into Sub-kingdoms by families, such as Conifers, Asters, and Solanaceae.

Universal Language (Also Called Non-Human Specific Words) in Everyday Speech

Universal Language uses expressions that *might* be used to describe a human experience of an emotion or a bodily sensation, but could also easily be used to describe the experience of some other substance in nature (such as minerals, plants, or animals). Often times these words will appear in the patient's descriptions and come across to the listener as "strange, rare and peculiar" ways of explaining something. Learning to hear this "Universal" language in your patient's everyday speech is essential to practicing the Sensation Method.

After identifying the Vital Expression, you will find that extracting these types of words, and asking the patient to describe them further, leads quickly to information about the Kingdom (plant, animal, mineral, etc) of the remedy needed. At certain points in the case Universal Language may describe actual *qualities* of the Source material of the remedy that is needed.

Listed below are a few examples, but the list is nearly endless.

Examples of Universal Language:
Hard
Attack
Stinging
Pressure
Floating
Heavy
Tight
Coiling
Tearing

Examples of *Human-Specific* (not Universal) Language*
Love
Busy
Jealous
Arguing
Affectionate
Schedule
Career
Rude
Nightmarish
Ugly
Headache
Autism

Note: We may associate words like "jealous" with snakes; and "career" with minerals; and "nightmarish" with a plant like Stramonium, but the words themselves are human specific, and do not indicate remedies from those Kingdoms unless combined with consistent usage of non-human specific words from the appropriate Kingdoms.

Levels

The Bombay Study Group has identified seven levels at which a patient may experience their complaint and from which they speak about those experiences. These levels can be seen as differing maps, highlighting various features of the same terrain (the patient's state). Gathering information from all levels helps the homeopath form a more complete picture of the patient's state. Previous methods tended to focus only on certain levels, such as fact or emotion.

The seven levels are:

1. Name (e.g., "Arthritis")

2. Fact (e.g., "Worse with motion")

3. Emotion (e.g., "It makes me depressed")

4. Delusion (image) (e.g., "It feels as if my joints are rusty and don't have enough oil")

5. Sensation (Kingdom) (e.g., "It's stiff and feels raw and grinding")

6. Energy (Source) (e.g., Patient makes a noise and gesture that describes the energy pattern, or uses quality words that describe the Source – "cccrrr….rough and bumpy, it moves slowly")

7. Potentiality—The blank slate upon which the pattern appears.

The Importance of the Chief Complaint

A patient's story is often times misleading. We have learned to rely on their description of the Chief Complaint for the following reasons:

- It represents the unbalanced Vital Force in its most current form.

- It is more likely to go directly to the Vital Expression.

- It is a direct experience, which points to the truth and the energy pattern that underlies the whole case.

- It is the central pillar of the case.

- It is like the tip of the iceberg in the case, an acute manifestation of the total state.

- It is a perfect holographic representation of the whole, a tiny part of the human being mirroring the totality.

- The patient wants the Chief Complaint cured.

How do we explore the Chief Complaint?

- By eliciting the raw experience or sensation from the Chief Complaint—not the common situation, emotions or unrelated delusions.
- By exploring the area where the body and the mind express the same phenomena (Vital Expression).
- By exploring the strange, rare, and peculiar within the main complaint.

Nonsense! The Importance of the Strange, Rare and Peculiar, and How it Fits with the Sensation Method.

All methods of homeopathy look for strange, rare and peculiar symptoms. However, in the Sensation Method, you will find yourself and your patient in a land where there is such a distillation of these odd details, that the "strange, rare and peculiar" will pop out to a degree rarely seen through more traditional casetaking. At this point in the case, patients will often comment, "This sounds like utter nonsense. I don't have any idea what I am talking about." Yet they can feel it has an accuracy that relates directly to their Vital Disturbance, and in fact, it relates directly to the Source of the remedy they need.

Hahnemann described the importance of focusing your attention on these details:

> "The more striking, singular, uncommon and peculiar (characteristic) signs
> and symptoms of the case of disease are chiefly and most solely to be kept in
> view; for it is more particularly these that very similar ones in the list of
> symptoms of the selected medicine must correspond to, in order to constitute it
> the most suitable for effecting the cure. The more general and undefined
> symptoms: loss of appetite, headache, debility, restless sleep, discomfort, and so
> forth, demand but little attention when of that vague and indefinite character,
> if they cannot be more accurately described, as symptoms of such a general
> nature are observed in almost every disease and from almost every drug."
> Organon §153:

Energy Patterns

Energy patterns are the shared qualities between a patient's remedy state and the substance in nature from which the corresponding remedy is made—including the substance's movement, color, sound, and life pattern. These energy patterns can often be seen in the patient's symptoms, gestures, tone, and general state. (The patterns themselves can also be described by the patient when she is speaking from the energy level—which is then called "Source language." See below.)

For example, people needing Mineral remedies from Row 4 of the Periodic Table often (but not always) use gestures that indicate movement from one place to another with some force. A person needing a Plant remedy that expands and contracts with moisture (such as a cactus) will experience symptoms and sensations of expansion and contraction and will unknowingly use gestures that mimic the expansion and contraction of the plant.

Source Language

In some cases, patients will describe the energy pattern they are experiencing so clearly and in such detail that, in retrospect, we can see that they were describing qualities of the Source material of the remedy that they needed. This is called "Source language." Images at other points in the case have often been confused for Source language. This manual will help you to differentiate between the two.

Hand Gestures as Expressions of Energy Patterns

Hand gestures are often sub-conscious, involuntary and often not noticed by the patient. The patient's hand gestures can be seen as non-verbal expressions of the energy pattern that is disturbing the patient, and which relates to the remedy that is needed. Homeopaths working in the Sensation Method must train themselves to keep their peripheral vision focused on the patient, even while taking notes, so that strong gestures are seen and noted.

Hand gestures are important when they are repetitive in various different situations described, and when they are strong and specific, rather than just a quick conversational gesture—though you should note all gestures, until you get a sense of whether the person is a *high* gesture type or a *low* gesture type

PART 3: HEARING THE VITAL EXPRESSION

Why Do We Need to Find the Vital Expression?

The Vital Expression can connect us directly to the information about which Kingdom the patient's remedy needs to be chosen from. It is only by probing the Vital Expression that we can clearly establish this. If you know when you have found an aspect of the Vital Expression, and you ask for more information about it, then you can clearly hear the Kingdom language and proceed from there to find the Sub-kingdom and qualities of the remedy.

Why Do We Need to Establish the Kingdom and Sub-kingdom?

One of the most common errors people make when using the Sensation Method is that they understand the energy pattern of the remedy, but they have not clearly identified the Kingdom and Sub-kingdom, and end up prescribing on the energy pattern and a random sampling of images that the patient used, which may or may not be a reflection of the Source. For example, one could have a case where the energy pattern is of something that starts off very contained, and then bursts out with a lot of violence and destruction, like a volcano, or a soda bottle, or an exploding bomb, or an animal charging out of its lair, etc.

Without knowing the Kingdom, the remedy could be a plant with a sensation of exploding and violence, such as Solanaceae, or it could be a mineral like Nitrogen. It could be an imponderable, like a Geyser, or it could be an animal that uses a quick burst of energy when going in for the kill, like a cheetah. Recently, we have seen many cases like this, where the remedy was prescribed by choosing one of the many images the patient used, and asking the patient to describe that image in detail, and then saying, "You see, this is Source language." These prescriptions can work sometimes, either by luck (that the homeopath happened to choose the right image to ask about), or because there is enough of a similarity in the energy pattern that the remedy functions for a time as a Simillimum, but after a few months or even a year, the prescription does not hold. The biggest problem with this sort of casetaking is that it is not replicable.

The patient may name a substance when it is the energy pattern they are trying to convey, not the substance itself. Many times, when you know the Kingdom, and Sub-kingdom from the Vital Expression, and the patient names a substance from another Kingdom, you can ask about this substance. The *name* of the thing is not important—it is the *qualities* they are trying to express. If the patient names a substance and it fits the Kingdom and Sub-kingdom, and when you ask about the qualities of this substance, everything still fits, then you can confidently prescribe this substance. Sometimes the patient names a substance and it is close to the prescription because it is in the same Sub-kingdom, but the qualities are slightly different so you will have to use the Materia Medica or Doctrine of

Signatures to confirm the exact substance. For example, the patient says Tiger, but from their descriptive Source words, and what you know about the remedy, they really need Lac Leoninum.

The Three Ways to Identify an Aspect of the Vital Expression in Your Case

1. A sensation or unusual expression is repeated in two or more unrelated areas.

> This could be two different physical complaints, or a physical and mental, mental and emotional, or physical and emotional complaint.

> For example, the patient says, "With the knee pain, I feel very stiff and I cannot move." She describes her problems with her mother-in-law, "I feel scared as if she is going to attack me. I feel extremely stiff and I just can't move." "Stiffness" and "cannot move" are part of the Vital Expression, in this case associated with both a local physical sensation and a sensation associated with an emotional state.

2. A sensation or unusual expression is repeated over and over without external probing, and is accompanied by a hand gesture.

> For example, a patient repeats over and over that his jealousy feels like breaking, burning and twisting. This is a strange, rare and peculiar way to describe jealousy and so "breaking, burning and twisting" could be an aspect of the Vital Expression.

> However, if you start to explore the Vital Expression with this method, you need to be sure you are not leading the patient to repeat themselves, and that the expression they use is not a common expression used in every day language. You should feel confident that what they say is actually their own internal expression.

> For example: "I need support in my life" repeated over and over could be a common expression, so be very cautious to choose "support" as a Vital Expression. The more strange, rare and peculiar the expressions, the more sure you will be that it is the Vital Expression.

3. A sensation or unusual expression is expressed in only one area but is accompanied by a powerful and spontaneous hand gesture and vocal emphasis.

> For example: In a very monotone patient, where there are very few gestures or intonations, he says it feels like "Whooosh!! *Down* the slide" and the sound is accompanied with a large movement of the arm. "Whooosh!!" could be an opening into the Vital Expression.

Another example, the patient growls while showing a strong gesture. The "growl" could be the Vital Expression.

The Vital Expression Can Manifest in the Chief Complaint in a Variety of Ways, Even Within the Same Case

The examples below are ways to begin to recognize the Vital Expression. You must be careful not to jump too quickly on a possible Vital Expression until you have confirmed it in one of the three ways:

1. Spontaneous expression repeated in two areas of the person's life and/or complaints

2. Very strong gesture or with a lot of energy, or

3. Spontaneous expression with gestures repeated over and over without direct questions about the expression. It is important to probe gently like, "Tell me more," and not extract out Universal Language and repeat it back to the patient until the Vital Expression is indicated strongly.

Examples:

- **Local sensations.** In Plant cases, the local sensations often *are* the Vital Expression. These patients tend to get frustrated with your questions early on, because to them, that's all there is. Generally in arthritis cases, words like "aching," "sore" and "tender" don't mean much because they are common and local symptoms of arthritis, but if those words keep coming and coming, it may be a Plant case with that sensation as the Vital Expression.

- **Modalities.** The Vital Expression can be expressed in the modality of the Chief Complaint. For example, the patient has rapid heart palpitations aggravated by any excitement. In further exploration of the case, the patient has a vivid imagination, racing thoughts, day dreams, and feels easily elated. These symptoms, which all relate to excitement and stimulation, may indicate a remedy from the Rubiaceae plant family such as Coffea. Excitement is the Vital Expression.

- **Physical manifestation of an emotional complaint.** The Chief Complaint can also be a mental or emotional complaint such as depression or anxiety. Then the questioning would need to elicit how it is experienced in the person's body and life, which will help to uncover the Vital Expression.

  For example, a patient comes with depression. You can ask how he experiences the depression. The patient may say that he experiences it in his body as "heaviness." He then goes on to say, as part of his description of the depression, "My life is a burden. My work load feels too heavy and relationships are cumbersome." Therefore the Vital Expression may have something to do with heaviness, like a burden.

- **Effect of Chief Complaint on the patient.** For example, a person has a dry cough that embarrasses him at work. He finds that because of this, he is incapable of achieving his goals. This could be the Vital Expression at the level of Emotion, but you don't know yet. So you ask, "Tell me more."

He says "I feel pressured by everything, my job, my wife, my knee… it's all pressure like I never got the frame of my house together." "Pressured" could be the Vital Expression, especially if accompanied with a strong gesture. The image of the house is at the Delusion level.

"Tell more…"

He says, "This pressure—it's something lacking in me, a void—I can't get from point A to point B. It's like I'm functioning as a dotted line." Now you know the level of Kingdom is about structure, indicating a Mineral remedy, because he is expressing his existence, "what is" for him is lacking—something between point A and point B. This is Universal Language of the Mineral Kingdom and indicates 4th Row (according to Dr. Andreas Holling's chart see Appendix for more details).

Another person says "This cough embarrasses me, it sounds gross, it attacks me, I have to hide it or I'll be shunned, and my survival depends on being part of the group at work." The Vital Expression could be "attacks me," especially if accompanied with a strong gesture. In this example, there are indications that it is an Animal remedy and that the animal is part of a group rather than a loner animal.

Caution: Don't mistake interests for Vital Expression: A patient who breeds pigeons will have a lot of energy talking about pigeons. Does this mean pigeons have something to do with his Vital Expression, or that he needs pigeon remedy? Maybe. You may have one patient who breeds pigeons who needs Pigeon remedy, but the next patient who breeds pigeons doesn't necessarily. The qualities and energy of the patient's state must be expressed at the Vital Expression, level of Kingdom and throughout the case.

PART 4: CASETAKING STEPS

In the actual process of casetaking, these are no rigidly fixed steps—rather, the process is somewhat fluid and sometimes overlaps from one area of a case to another. This lack of clarity from one phase of casetaking to the next has led to confusion between Source language and Image/Delusional language.

Although it is somewhat artificial, it can be helpful to look at the process as a series of steps, with the understanding that one must gather certain materials from the patient at each stage of the case, before the next stage's information becomes relevant or useful. Therefore, we have broken the process down into a series of steps in order to clarify what to look for at each stage, and at what points you should narrow down your questioning in order to get information about Kingdom, Sub-kingdom and Source.

STEP 1: Explore the Chief Complaint
until you get a clear sense of the Vital Expression

What you need to do at this step:

Just ask and listen

- Ask, "What is bothering you?" "What is your main problem?" or "What can I help you with?"

- Ask the patient to describe their own experience of the Chief Complaint.

- Ask open-ended questions such as, "Tell me more about that." And, "What is the experience of that?"

- Do not focus on a specific word or gesture until you are sure you have found an aspect of the Vital Expression.

- Leave plenty of time for the patient to answer. If they are staying on track, do not interrupt them with another question until they say, "that's it." A simple "tell me more" will support the patient to keep talking.

Keep the patient focused on the main complaint and sensations related to it

- If the patient diverts to the emotional sphere in the very beginning of the case, then bring him back to the Chief Complaint. If the Chief Complaint is an emotional or situational complaint, ask the patient to describe *how they experience it*, not what is happening or why.

- There are situations where the patient spontaneously goes to a dream or relates their Chief Complaint to an intense time in their lives. If this happens, then you must follow the patient, and oftentimes this leads directly to the Vital Expression. If not, then ask the patient to go back to the Chief Complaint and tell you more.

- Oftentimes the patient gives many details about When and Why the Chief Complaint happened. What you need to find out is: *what is the experience* of this problem for the patient.

- Sometimes you must be firm, if the patient is continually just telling their story. Gently interrupt the patient, repeat the last descriptive words, and ask for a further elaboration of the experience.

- If, after several questions, the patient does not easily describe their main complaint in terms of a sensation, ask them how that experience feels in the body.

- Many times you will need to ask the patient to describe specific physical sensations when they are in a "worst case" scenario of their problem—as opposed to how they are feeling at the moment.

- If there is a peculiar modality, ask about that.

Gradually start mirroring back to the patient any Universal Language and gestures he is using.

- Once you have a sense of the whole pattern of the main complaint, or if the patient says that is all there is to tell, repeat back *the whole list* of Universal Language (or *non-human specific*) words he has used and ask him to tell you more. For example: "You said your headache is splitting, exploding, and pressurized. Can you tell me more?"

- Sometimes stop the patient while he is gesturing and ask him what the gesture means—especially if it is very intense or repeated numerous times. You will want to wait before jumping in and asking too soon, because the patient may just look blankly at you. If the person has exhausted most of what they can say about the Chief Complaint and you've seen the gesture has some energy, then ask.

- When an intense gesture is discovered, and if the description continues to have consistency and energy, then explore further. This may lead to the Vital Expression. The Vital Expression will be confirmed in Step 2. If you have discovered the Vital Expression, the case will open easily; if it fizzles out, then you need to repeat Step 1 until you clearly identify the Vital Expression.

In cases where someone easily uses Delusional Language, then be cautious and wait to repeat Universal Language until you hear the same expressions repeated often.

- The best question throughout Step 1 is simply "tell me more." The more you can stay in the space of the unprejudiced observer and level of Potentiality, where you are open to the spontaneous and strange, rare and peculiar, the more you will observe and understand where you are in the case.

If the patient seems uncomfortable or hesitant:

- Acknowledge and support the patient through the casetaking process.

- Reassure the patient and give a short explanation of the method.

- Explain that there are no wrong answers, to say whatever comes into their head.

- Say: "I'm going to ask the same question over and over again, not because I don't understand your answer, but because each time I ask the same question, you give me a little more information, which helps me to understand your case."

- You can tell the patient: "You have explained the situation very well, and now what I need to know is how you *experience* the situation."

- Say: "You are doing great. I understand that the pain is (sticking, poking, hard). Please tell me more…"

- Ask: "How does the Chief Complaint affect your life? What does the Chief Complaint mean for you in your life? What does it stop you from doing? What problems does it create?"

What you are looking for in this step:

FACTS: Gather as many facts as you will need about the symptoms of the main complaint early on in this stage, because as you progress to the other stages, you will want to steer the patient away from facts, emotions, and stories, and into the images, sensations, and energy patterns of the case—which will be unfamiliar territory for most patients. Asking about facts early on in the case also establishes a level of trust for the patient—by showing that you are truly interested in understanding their symptoms.

LOCAL SENSATIONS: The first sensations expressed by the client may not be the Vital Expression. However, in terms of understanding and confirming the remedy later, it is important to understand the local sensations precisely. Ask more about the local sensations until the patient cannot go any further, or the patient repeats images about the same thing.

- INTENSITY: Note descriptive words that carry some *intensity* through intonation of the voice, or that are accompanied by a strong gesture. Note gestures that have intensity and stand out from minor hand movements or from a non-gesturing patient.

- REPETITION: Look out for *repeated* hand and facial gestures, and more generalized body language, as well as repeated words or phrases.

- UNIVERSAL LANGUAGE (non-human specific language): note words that are non-human specific, such as pressure, clawing, tight, vibrating, attack, floating, etc.

- PATTERNS: Note patterns of words that may be related (e.g. they all sound mineral-like or animal-like, or expressive of a similar sensation, even if they are not all the same.)

- STRANGE, RARE AND PECULIAR: Pay attention to any gesture or word that seems out of context to what is spoken. For example, the patient says, "I feel love" but clenches her fist.

What is not Strange, Rare and Peculiar?

You need to constantly question your analysis, especially when it comes to strange, rare and peculiar symptoms. Here are a few examples of language which is not strange, rare or peculiar, which, if used to classify, would lead to poor prescriptions:

- A mother saying that she would grieve more for her child than her husband is not strange, rare and peculiar and would not necessarily indicate a Mammal.

- A man saying that he is not functioning well at his job is not strange, rare and peculiar, and would not necessarily indicate a Mineral case or a remedy from the Kali row.

MIASMATIC CLUES: (not confirmation, which usually occurs in the next step)

- Look for the pace and depth of the problem.
- Look at the patient's response or attitude or coping mechanism.
- If there seems to be no Vital Expression other than miasmatic words, it may be a Nosode case, though these are rare, so keep looking.

Remember, the sensation becomes general and is possibly the Vital Expression when it is:

- Experienced in the same way in another location other than the Chief Complaint; in other words, the client spontaneously gives the same expression when speaking about the Chief Complaint and some other complaint. This is particularly true if one complaint is mental and the other physical.

- Expressed through repetitive and/or intense gestures, or

- Experienced with a lot of energy accompanied with a hand gesture.

- Repeated over and over, when asked open-ended questions—without you asking them about that particular word.

STEP 2: Exploring the Vital Expression and determining the Kingdom, Sub-kingdom and miasm.

GOALS: The Vital Expression is the doorway into the language of Kingdom. Therefore, the goals at this step are to:

1. "Dissociate" the patient from their local complaints and emotions (i.e., You ask the patient to stop talking about themselves and their own story, and you focus and note the Universal Language and gestures that are emerging from the Vital Expression.)

2. Get the patient to describe their Vital Expression.

3. Keep the questions very simple—do not use extra words. Simple phrases like "Tell me more" or "What is Your Experience?" are best.

4. Understand what in the patient's description is Universal Language and therefore Kingdom related.

5. Refine that description of the Vital Expression to understand Sub-kingdom and miasm at the level of Kingdom.

What the Homeopath needs to do:

- When you think you have identified the Vital Expression, start repeating back the words of the Vital Expression and showing the gestures in order for the patient to give you more Universal Language (non-human-specific words), and miasmatic expressions. For example: "Tell me more about this sensation of heaviness. Describe 'heaviness', what are you showing with your hands?"

- Listen for words that may indicate a specific Kingdom. If the Vital Expression is appearing as an issue of heaviness, with a gesture of pushing down, do they define this heaviness as an issue of structure and function ("heavy, useless, unable to do anything, totally non-productive")? As a sensitivity and its opposite ("I feel pressed down, I want to spread out and move, I'd rather be floating") or as an issue of survival and victimization ("It's like being held down by someone much larger than me, like being frozen in fear")?

- As this Kingdom language emerges, continue to repeat back the Vital Expression *as well as* any sensation words and other universal words that occur. "Spreading, growing, expanding—use more words."

- Ask the patient to describe any gestures they make as they refine their description of the Vital Expression. It is usually better to ask after the gesture is repeated over and over, or has intense energy with it.

- Tell them "I don't want to hear any more about your ear/head/back etc. I only want to know about this spreading, growing, expanding and this thing you are showing with your hands."

- There are times when you will need to dissociate the patient in order to understand the Kingdom and Sub-kingdom from the Vital Expression. There is more information about how to use this technique in Step 3: *Going to Source*. When you are sure of the Vital Expression but are not sure of the Kingdom and Sub-kingdom, ask the patient to tell you just about the Vital Expression, not about themselves, their complaint or their situation. It can be from the imagination, just whatever comes to mind—and in this way you will be able to confirm the Kingdom, Sub-kingdom and possibly spontaneously go to Source language. In this case, if you get the Kingdom and Sub-kingdom, you can repeat the process again to take the patient deeper so that you will have more Source language at the level of Energy, following the directions of Step 3: *Going to Source*.

How to Use Images*:* Images or Delusional Language will frequently be used at this level, which is fine, but remember that what you are looking for is not the image itself. If the patient uses delusion/image language, such as metaphors and similes, keep asking them about the Vital Expression words, as well as any universal words that occur in their image. Do not ask them to tell you more about the image itself.

For example, if they say "This feeling of everything gushing out is like a barrel that is overflowing," then you say, "Good, tell me more about gushing out and overflowing." *Don't* ask them about barrels.

Ask about the verbs, adjectives or adverbs, rather than the nouns—that will help you to stay with the energy pattern, rather than having them describe the image itself. The image is a name of a symbol and actually is not important in this

process. It is the *experience* and *qualities* of the image you want to know—
especially when you have identified the Vital Expression.

What you are looking for in this step:

- KINGDOM
- SUB-KINGDOM
- MIASM

KINGDOM:

Is the Vital Expression experienced as a problem of sensitivity, survival, or
structure/function?

Once you have found the Vital Expression, and you ask the person to describe it
more fully, they will start to define the Kingdom as a way to describe the Vital
Expression. This will be expressed in Universal or non-human-specific
Language:

- *Plant: The sensation is all within me.* Vital Expression, when explored in the
  Plant Kingdom, will be expressed as *sensitivity and reactivity* to a certain
  group of (often opposite) sensations. The sensation and its opposite will
  be repeated throughout most Plant cases at the level of
  Kingdom/Sensation. The patient will spontaneously use the opposite as a
  way to define the sensation without your having to *ask* for the opposite,
  for example "tight is when something is not loose, it's tight and clenched,
  not loose and relaxed." If you need to ask for the opposite, it probably
  isn't a Plant case.

- *Animal: The sensation is outside of me.* Vital Expression, when explored in an
  Animal Kingdom case, will be an issue of *survival, competition, attractiveness,
  split within oneself and victim vs. aggressor* at the level of Kingdom.

- *Mineral: The sensation is about me.* Vital Expression, when explored in a
  Mineral Kingdom case, is expressed as a *problem of (lack of, or necessity to
  reach, or regain) structure, function, capacity, performance, and existence* at the level
  of Kingdom.

- *Fungi:* Our understanding of the fungi as a Kingdom is just emerging.

- *Nosodes (Monera):* Vital Expression, when explored in the Monera
  Kingdom, is expressed as a miasm (coping mechanism) which is repeated
  in all spheres of the case without any other theme or expression. For
  example, if, in all of the expressions of the Vital Expression from the
  patient, all you elicit is the need to escape, a feeling of "I can't breathe,"
  and the need to change continuously, you are looking at the coping

strategy of the Tubercular miasm, and possibly the prescription would be Tuberculinum. Be aware that miasms are present in all cases, whereas the expression of the miasm is consistent and intense in a nosode case.

- *Imponderables:* The imponderable remedies (such as Electricitas, Positronium, Sun) are mostly an unknown territory; however, when a patient describes in specific language a substance that is an imponderable, you can consider it for a prescription. The imponderables will sometimes use Source language that sounds mineral-like, but there will be no corresponding issues of function, structure, or existence. The Vital Expression will be explored beyond time and space at the level of Kingdom.

Caution: Don't try to determine the Kingdom from just one or two words. It is the whole expression of the Universal Language that indicates a Kingdom. With experience, you will easily identify Kingdoms. In the beginning, it is useful to seek review of your cases from homeopaths experienced with this method, because many mistakes occur at this stage. We tend to look at what is familiar, ignore what doesn't fit, and make assumptions. In some cases, there are subtle distinctions between the Kingdoms, and in other cases it can be quite obvious.

If the Kingdom is not easily confirmed:

When the Vital Expression is well-identified, the case will open easily. It should not be a struggle. If asking about the Vital Expression does not lead to Kingdom language, the words you chose to ask about probably are *not* an aspect of the Vital Expression—you may have jumped too quickly on a local sensation or non-universal, *human*-specific language. If this happens, you should go back to the main complaint and reexamine it following the procedures of Step 1, or take another complaint through all the Steps.

If the patient jumps too quickly to Energy level and expresses Source language (describes the qualities of the remedy they need) without confirming the Vital Expression or Kingdom, then you need to go back to Step 1, confirm the Vital Expression, and repeat back the Universal Language to the patient while avoiding repetition of the quality words of the possible substance. In this way you will confirm the Vital Expression and listen for more Universal Language to confirm the Kingdom and Sub-kingdom; then, if all the information fits, you can repeat back the Source language and understand the remedy better from the way the patient describes it. This situation of jumping to Source language too soon can happen with patients who are highly intuitive or who need drug-type remedies.

SUB-KINGDOM:

The Sub-kingdom is expressed as a pattern of information within the Kingdom language. Our understanding of these patterns and ability to match them to Sub-kingdoms is being further refined as this work is advancing.

In order to explore the Sub-kingdom, you must note all the Universal, non-human-specific words that are repeated by the patient. Many times it is very obvious what the patient is describing; sometimes it is very difficult, and this is where further research may be necessary—through books, computer programs, on the internet, and/or with colleagues. In the section on analyzing Kingdoms and Sub-kingdoms later, we have explained this further and suggested useful resources for more information.

Exploring the Sub-kingdom: Possible Plant Case

If the initial Kingdom language is pointing to the Plant Kingdom, you need to confirm that the Vital Expression at the level of Kingdom is persistent. Oftentimes, there are consistently opposite sensations, which the patient spontaneously offers up as a way to describe the sensation. For example, if you ask about "loose," the person says "it is loose, not tight, not squeezing," At that point, the homeopath needs to understand the sensation in all its permutations. For example, many Plant families have a sensation of shock, but by persisting with the questioning about shock, one can understand the active and passive reactions, and what the shock is associated with—is it associated with pain? with injury? with a sudden attack? These sensations would help to differentiate the Papaveracea, Compositae, and Umbelliferae families. (See "Sankaran's Schema," "Insight into Plants Vol. 1-3," and "Vital Quest" software to better understand these sub-families.)

When the sensations of a Plant family are clearly one of the Plant families charted, then it is necessary to understand the miasm so that you can use the chart and find the remedy under a specific Plant family and miasm. If there seem to be Plant sensations that are not charted, then it is possible to use rubrics and Materia Medica to find the remedy based on these sensations, as well as any Source information to support your prescription.

Exploring the Sub-kingdom in a Possible Animal Case

If the initial Kingdom language is pointing to an Animal case, the homeopath should then probe the Vital Expression to elicit the Animal Sub-kingdom to understand the patterns and gestures that will give the particular animal group and specific Animal remedy.

Once in the Sub-kingdom, feed back more Sub-kingdom language, patterns, and gestures until the patient gives enough qualities to confirm the specific Animal remedy, which can later be confirmed in dreams and through other physical complaints, fears, generals, etc. Sometimes it is necessary to probe hobbies, books, movies, etc.—anything that excites the person at the delusional and emotional levels, to confirm the prescription. Sometimes the miasm will help to determine the animal group (i.e. Tubercular miasm could be an insect, Sycotic miasm could be a mammal, etc.), but there are many exceptions.

In Animal cases, you will usually hear of lot of different Universal Language—a complex pattern emerges. At times it will sound like what is being described is contradictory. The life of an animal has many stages and activities, such as the birthing, nourishing, reproductive, dying, etc. The language from the Vital Expression will reflect this complexity, and you just need to follow the patient and watch all the patterns emerge until it is clear if this is a mammal, a bird, an insect, etc.

Exploring the Sub-kingdom: Possible Mineral Case

If the patient's language is indicating a Mineral case, the next step is to find the Sub-kingdom—the line and/or column in the periodic table. You also need to understand how many themes there are in the case—if there is more than one theme, this may indicate a salt or compound.

With Mineral cases, it is often easiest to find the Sub-kingdom by letting the patient drop back into Delusion language and noting the themes that have been identified by Scholten, Sankaran and others. However, other methods of analyzing Minerals are emerging. See the section on Sub-kingdoms below for more information.

Caution: "It ain't over till it's over…"

At any point during or after taking a case, you may suddenly realize you are on the wrong track, and have misidentified the Kingdom or Sub-kingdom. We cannot stress enough how important it is to keep your mind open to this possibility at all times. You should always be listening for what *doesn't* fit with your current understanding of the case. Those details should never be ignored, and must be fully explored and understood before settling on a prescription. Always keep the attitude of: "This sounds at this point like a Mineral case, but what else could it be?"

MIASM: Probe the Vital Expression and, in addition to the Kingdom and Sub-kingdom, the miasm will become apparent. The Kingdom language and miasm are two sides of the same coin. When you ask about how the patient experiences their Vital Expression, the patient should give miasm language. Sometimes the miasm will be indicated from hints throughout the case. Language indicating miasm will often include references to other miasms that are closely related—for example Leprosy Miasm is related to Syphilitic, and so you will hear both. Patient's needing Syphilitic Miasm remedies, however, will not generally use

miasmatic terms associated with Leprosy Miasm (such as dirty, disgusting, etc.)
See the section on Miasms for more information.

STEP 3: Going to the Source

The goal at this step is to help the patient access the place where they can
describe the qualities of the substance that is needed (the "Source").

What the homeopath needs to do:

Ask for Qualities: Repeat the Vital Expression and the Kingdom and Sub-
kingdom words that have occurred, with the gestures, and ask the patient to
describe qualities: movement, color, texture, sounds—anything that comes to
mind.

Feed back their energy: Be sure to use the same intonation and quality of
energy that the person expresses. For example, if the person speaks softly and
slowly, then you should repeat the words in the same rhythm, with the same
gestures and posture. Or, if he states things aggressively and leans forward while
telling you his experiences, then you do the same. Keep mirroring what the
patient does in front of you.

Keep yourself out of the picture: Only repeat the words of the patient—do not
use your own expressions, or tie the words into sentences, and definitely don't
add your comments or explanations of the meaning of these words.

It is fine, however, to briefly explain where you are at in the process. For
example: "I understand that these words (list the words of the patient) are your
Vital Expression and that this is an expression of your deeper state. There are
several remedies that express these qualities, so now I need you to go to the next
level to help me differentiate which would be the best remedy." Then be sure to
encourage and acknowledge how well the patient is doing so far.

Keep them out of the picture, too: If the patient starts to go back into their
story or symptoms, generally you should stop them. Sometimes patients will
backtrack if it is uncomfortable for them to stay at this level of Energy. On the
other hand, if the patient is not an incessant story-teller, and spontaneously
wants to tell you something significant about their life, or a dream, or a
childhood incident, then you definitely want to listen, because at this level,
information that comes up spontaneously may relate directly to the Source.

Ask them to just be with it: If the level of Energy is not easily and
spontaneously happening in front of you, you can take a pause: ask the patient to
loosen his jaw, take several deep breaths, and close his eyes if he is comfortable
with this; then, repeat back the words and gestures of the Kingdom and Sub-
kingdom. Then wait.

Encourage non-verbal expressions: It can also be helpful to ask the patient to draw or show you in some way what comes to mind when you repeat all those words. Tell them it does not have to make sense, to say whatever comes to mind—that it can be completely from the imagination, or just make a doodle, etc.

Find what doesn't fit: When a substance is named, be sure to listen to what does not fit, and ask more about those qualities. It is common for people speaking at this level to be able to describe a substance and not be able to name it, because they are experiencing the substance on the Energy level, not on the Name level.

Don't push them to name the substance: If they do name a substance, and it all fits, then you can trust the naming of the substance. If they don't name a substance, don't push them to name it, or you may take them back to the Fact and/or Delusion level and away from the actual Source qualities.

Write down the Universal Language and Vital Expression: Sometimes you need to write down all the words spoken that are the Vital Expression, Kingdom and Sub-kingdom, even possibly Source words, and ask the patient to add more and explain more; and then ask them again to talk about this Universal Language, not about them or their situation. Many times, they'll go back to talk about their complaints, which is fine—but you want to listen for more of the Universal Language, and keep repeating those expressions back so that you hear more and more of the Sub-kingdom and Source language. In many cases, it is worth staying on this level of Energy to get as much information as you can. Don't stop too early.

What the homeopath needs to understand:

- Be aware that images may still occur at this Energy level. Just because the patient names a substance, it still may not be the correct remedy. That's—because when a patient connects to the universal information, it is through the *qualities* of the substance, not the *name* of the substance. Ask them to describe the qualities, not the name.

- Once a person goes to the symbol or name of the remedy, they may no longer connect to the substance itself.

- Synchronicities and spontaneous changes of direction in conversation at this point are often significant:: a light bulb blows out, a toilet overflows, or the person says, totally out of the blue, "You know, I am really into raising pigs."

- Source language in Mineral cases is intriguing, but often not helpful in identifying which mineral someone needs, since most homeopaths are not that familiar with the subtle differences in physical properties of minerals. However, the Source language can be very helpful in confirming a prescription, once it has been chosen. For example, a heavy metal has a different quality than a gas or radioactive substance.

- **Caution**: Source language should not be the basis for your prescription. The prescription needs to be firmly grounded in the Kingdom and Sub-kingdom language the patient has given from the Vital Expression. Source language should only serve to refine and confirm your prescription.

Caution about Drug Remedy Types: People needing Drug remedies (which can be from any Kingdom) can quickly channel universal information because they are in a drug state. This is Source language, but it is not *their* Source language. Don't let them do that until you are 100 percent sure of the Vital Expression, Kingdom, and Sub-kingdom.

STEP 4: Confirm the prescription in other areas

The goal of Step 4 is to make sure your prescription is accurate and not just "hit or miss." Before you begin on this step, make sure you know that you have found the Vital Expression, and have understood the Kingdom, Sub-kingdom, miasm and Source.

What the homeopath needs to do:

- **Ask about other areas:** Confirm the prescription by asking about other areas of the patient's life—exploring other symptoms in detail, asking about dreams, fears, etc. This is especially important if the case went very quickly through all the steps. You want to be sure that you find the Vital Expression in another area of the patient's life—another part of the same iceberg. Be sure that the same Kingdom is confirmed, then the Sub-kingdom and then Source language.

- **Make sure it hangs together:** Make sure all the pieces of the case hang together and fit your understanding of the Kingdom, Sub-kingdom, Source, and miasm. Check the Materia Medica and make sure that the Delusions, Generals, and Strange, Rare and Peculiars match with the proving—or if it is a less-well known remedy, then to a remedy well-known in the same Sub-kingdom.

- **Look for what doesn't fit:** While probing other areas of the patient's life, you should be looking for things that do not fit with the rest of the case. If you find something, you MUST follow it, and try to understand it—often it will be the most important piece of information. It could change your entire understanding of the case.

- **If things don't fit, don't get discouraged.** Many times, if you are on the right track and you keep your mind open, even if you think something doesn't fit, you will keep probing and then find the original expressions return from the most unusual places. For example, in a successful case of Positronium, the patient referred to the qualities of "before time," "ageless," etc., and then spontaneously brought up the image of an octopus with tentacles in the sea. Clearly this would indicate a problem, but as the case unfolded, the same theme of the pre-time, pre-existence repeated itself—confirming the Mineral/Imponderable Kingdom and not Animal Kingdom language. In this situation, the octopus is an image from the Delusion level, and only by going deeper were the Kingdom, Sub-kingdom and Source get reconfirmed.

- **Check your Repertory:** It is always a good idea to do a brief repertorization of the key points to make sure there isn't another obvious remedy that fits even better, and which you may have completely overlooked in your enthusiasm. The Sensation Method can be an intoxicating whirlwind of information for the practitioner, and sometimes you get carried away with your ideas—often based on an image the patient used—and your desire to have a great Source case.

- **Check your Materia Medica:** If the remedy is a well-proven remedy, the pathology should fit with what you read in the Materia Medica. If the remedy is a common remedy and you can't find most of the person's symptoms in the Materia Medica, and/or if the main pathology associated with the remedy isn't present in the case (e.g., bleeding in a Crotalus case, cramping in a cuprum case), you should proceed carefully. It's certainly possible you still have the right remedy, but the prognosis should drop, and you should take the time to reread and rethink the case before giving the remedy.

- **Check other sources:** If the remedy is not a well-proven remedy, or if you have a case with a clear Sub-kingdom but no Source (e.g., you know it's a spider but you don't know which one), this is the time to do a search on Google, or in your library of natural history books, to try to match up the energy patterns, qualities, and Source language with the substance in nature. If you click on "Images" on Google, you can see pictures of whatever you are searching for. Wikipedia can also be helpful as a relatively concise (though not always accurate) reference on many substances. Programs like Vital Quest, and homeopathy books like "Prisma," are starting to do some of this pattern-matching work for us as well.

- **Prescribe the remedy.** When everything fits, you can prescribe the remedy.

What the homeopath needs to understand:

- Experienced homeopaths working in the Sensation Method use pattern matching to recognize the Kingdom and Sub-kingdom, but be very careful of using your personal Rolodex to match what you think the patient is saying to something you think you know. Stay open and try not to think too much. Allow it to unfold. If you keep your mind open, the patient will give you everything you need.

- If, at the end of the case, you are not sure of the Kingdom or Sub-kingdom, you are better off analyzing the case using keynotes and rubrics, rather than trying to guess the remedy based on the imagery and Universal Language the patient used. There is nothing wrong with going back to older methods in a case that is too difficult. Use the method that is most likely to help this particular patient.

- Know that you don't know.

- It's okay to bring the patient back in for further interviewing if necessary.

- Ask for help if you are really uncertain. This is where working with colleagues who have an understanding of the Sensation Method can help you to recognize where you may have gone astray, or not gone deep enough. You also may have ended up in a realm of remedies you don't know much about, but which another colleague may know more about—or is able to refer you to someone who has this knowledge. Watch natural history programs on TV. Cultivate relationships with chemists, botanists, and zoologists!

In general, the homeopath should be more interested in:

- Universal Language (non-human specific words)
- Words that occur along with gestures
- Words that are out of context
- Words spoken after a long pause
- Gestures that are repeated
- Gestures with intensity
- Gestures out of context
- Patterns of energy
- Sounds and gestures combined to illustrate something
- Something unexpected or unusual that happens

Over time, you will develop a keener perception of recognizing energy and energy patterns, and develop an ear for Universal Language and the Vital Expression through casetaking and watching cases taken using this method.

Common Pitfalls of Casetaking

- Jumping too quickly into the case
- Choosing only one word to explore
- Confusing a sensation that is local (Fact level) with one that is general (Vital Expression)
- Using a bypass when not needed
- Confusing images with Source
- Confusing level of Kingdom/Sensation with level of Energy
- Not identifying the Vital Expression before determining the Kingdom, Sub-kingdom and Source
- Ignoring what you don't know
- Overly encouraging the patient to describe aspects that you associate with a certain remedy, which overemphasizes that aspect of the case in a way that didn't naturally unfold
- Filling in your ideas of what the substance must be from Source language without following the Vital Expression and confirming the Kingdom and Sub-kingdom

PART 5: SUCCESSFUL NAVIGATION THROUGH THE LEVELS

Levels as Overlapping Maps

Using the levels to understand where you are in the case is another way to look at the process of casetaking. All levels exist at the same time, like overlapping maps of an area. In your casetaking, you can zoom in and look at a particular level at a particular point in the case. When you do that, you are extracting information from the case at that level, but the other levels are still there. You may be looking at a street-sign map, which is equivalent to the Fact level, but you could zoom in and look at an emotional map of the same area when you are ready to, simply by asking the patient "how do you feel emotionally when that (fact) is happening?"

No matter what they are talking about, or where you are in the case, you can ask the patient a question to help see things from a different level. For example,

- When you are looking for Kingdom information, it's best to ask the patient to focus on the Kingdom/Sensation level. What you are aiming for is to get them using 80 percent Universal Language.

- When you are looking for Source information, you are asking them to use more quality words than factual, emotional, delusional, image or sensation words; therefore you are asking them to speak from the Energy level.

The Seven Levels

- **Level 1—Name**: Diagnosis, e.g., "Migraine."

- **Level 2—Fact**: Details of the illness or patient's life, e.g., "It happens at 3 p.m. It hurts on the left side only."

- **Level 3—Emotion**: Emotions experienced as a result of the main complaint, e.g., "It makes me really upset and frustrated."

- **Level 4—Delusion (or Image)**: Metaphors and images used to describe emotions or situations, e.g., "It's as if my head was a block of wood stuck in a vise."

- **Level 5—Kingdom (or Sensation)**: Universal Language of Sensation. The Kingdom and Sub-kingdom is determined at this level ideally from the Vital Expression. For example, "The pressure keeps getting tighter and tighter and tighter. It's crushing."

- **Level 6—Energy (or Source)**: The expression of the Source itself is expressed here through speed, shape, direction, color, and sound, gestures and noises like pfffff, zzzzzzzzzz, or sighing. It is here that the qualities of the substance are revealed as Source language. For example, "It's hot, it moves up and out with a lot of power."

- **Level 7—Potentiality**: The blank slate. The space where anything can manifest. Where the practitioner's mind should be. The unprejudiced observer.

Learn what you can about one level before moving onto the next

You need to extract out all the language, especially the Universal Language, you will need at the level you are in before moving to another level. Once you understand the level being explored, the patient will often move to another level more easily. The mirroring or repeating the Universal Language encourages the patient to use more words that will tell you the Kingdom and Sub-kingdom.

It is important to be aware that the client will express signs and language not only of the level they are currently focused on, but also of the levels before and after that. For example, at the level of Delusion, the client will also express some emotions, sensations, Kingdom and Source language. However, most of their description will be in the form of images and metaphors.

Different Pathways

The patient can follow various routes and focus on language from different levels, and should not be interrupted even as the case becomes clearer and clearer for you. Just keep listening for the Vital Expression, so that if the case stalls or needs prodding, you can pick it up from the Vital Expression. As long as the patient is moving easily from concentrating on one level to another, you can simply follow along even if the patient is jumping to different levels and back again.

For example: the patient's narrative may travel from Name to Fact to Emotion to Delusion to Kingdom/Sensation to Energy. Or sometimes from Fact to Kingdom/Sensation, and then to Delusion, then to Emotion, then Delusion, and finally back to Kingdom/Sensation. That is fine – just keep listening for the Vital Expression, without interrupting, because...

Patients will often express language from many levels but are most comfortable at one level. Or they may use language almost entirely from one particular level with only very slight hints of the other levels.

The levels of Name, Fact and Emotion are levels that do not need to be explored too deeply, as long as you understand the key points of the case, and have identified the Vital Expression. If the patient goes directly from Name, Fact or

Emotion to another level, there is no need to bring the patient back *if you have found the Vital Expression*—better to pursue the other levels of Kingdom/Sensation and Energy. If you need more factual details you can always ask about them at the end of the case, which can also be helpful to ground the person after an intense casetaking experience.

What to do if you get stuck at a certain level

Not all patients will flow easily from one level to another. Many cases will have a fixation at a specific level—in particular, at the level of Fact, Emotion or Delusion. When the client gets stuck at a particular level, then a new approach is needed to take the patient to a deeper level.

It is extremely important to encourage the patient at this point and explain what you are doing. You can tell them that they have done a great job telling you how they are feeling emotionally and about their situation, and that in order to give them a remedy, you need to understand their experience on some other levels—such as images of what it is like, and the sensations in the body.

You can also explain that there are many remedies for migraines (or whatever their Chief Complaint is), and that in order to distinguish which is the best, you need to understand how they experience their migraine on all different levels—factually, emotionally, in images, sensations, etc. When given encouragement, most people will relax and be able to continue on. The patient needs to feel like a partner in the process not someone being cross examined about their problems.

You want to establish a strong rapport with your patient without being overly sympathetic (don't use phrases such as "I know how hard it must have been…"). It is much more direct to match the tone, cadence, and intensity, and mimic their gestures in order to have the patient's full commitment to reveal their Source remedy to you.

1. Level of Name

Pathology: At the level of Name, the patient names the pathology; for example, arthritis, cirrhosis or asthma. Do not forget to ask about all their diagnoses, as some patients will skip right over any that are not their Chief Complaint. This information is helpful when confirming a remedy in the homeopathic literature, and obviously necessary when adding to our databases of cured cases of different pathologies.

Some patients are inordinately focused on details of the diagnosis, and whether or not it was the correct diagnosis—referring to the fact that this doctor called it this, and that doctor called it that, etc. *When the focus of the conversation is on the name of the diagnosis or illness, we say we are at the Name level.*

Questions to ask at the level of Name:

- What can I help you with?

- I'd like to start by having you list off all the things that are bothering you.

- Can you tell me what diagnoses you have received for these problems?

Questions to Ask to Move to the Next Level

After the client has fully explained the pathology, ask the following questions in order to move to the next level. *If there are many different complaints, be sure to ask which one is bothering her the most:*

- What is bothering you the most?

- Describe the problem.

- What is your experience of this problem?

- How does it affect you?

- How does it affect your life?

2. Level of Fact

Level of Fact as a base of information: At this level, the patient describes the various details of the problem or their story. *When the focus of the conversation is on these factual details, we say we are at the level of Fact.* This is the level where the symptoms of the Chief Complaint are identified. You need to understand the factual details completely, have them qualified as much as possible, and get all the peculiarities. This information is invaluable and forms the basis of information to confirm the various aspects that come up later in the case. Most of this basic case information can also be gathered at the end of the case if it is not spontaneously given at the beginning.

Local sensations at Fact level: At the Fact level, we have to understand the local sensations from the Chief Complaint very precisely, and then see how these local sensations become general, which will help to identify the Vital Expression. (Hearing sensation words at this point does not mean you are at the level of Kingdom and does not help to confirm the Kingdom.) Remember, do not let go of the Chief Complaint.

What to do while you are here: The homeopath needs to ask what the problem is, have it qualified and then find out the peculiars. For example, it is a pain in the knee (what), worse with motion (qualified) and better from eating cucumbers (peculiar). At this level a local phenomenon can become general (the Vital Expression), when it is experienced in the same way in another location other than the Chief Complaint.

Take careful notes as to the facts of the case. At the same time, pay attention to any emotions, delusions and sensations. Do not jump on any particular word until you are *sure* of the Vital Expression. Simply keep asking the patient to tell you more. Observe the energy, the gestures and characteristic expressions that come up while describing the Chief Complaint.

If the patient gets lost with too many details, take her back to the Chief Complaint. If the patient diverts to emotional aspects, bring her back to the Chief Complaint again until the Fact level is exhausted.

Once the Fact level has been exhausted, if any word, gesture, or image is repeated, shows intense energy, or is totally out of context, follow the lead of the words or images into the next level. If you haven't noticed anything repetitive or intense, then ask about another symptom, or about the emotions associated with the symptoms, which will help you see anything that is generalized between two symptoms or between mind and body.

Questions to ask to move to another level:

- "How do you feel about this (complaint), or when this (complaint) happens?" *(This question will take you to Emotion level, if they are stuck at Fact level.)*

- "Describe more about… (intense or repeated Universal Language)…— not your complaints themselves, but just the experience of (x)." "Leave yourself aside, and just describe (x)." *(This question will usually take you to Delusion or Kingdom/Sensation level.)*

- Describe more about this gesture. What are you showing with your hands? *Be sure to show the patient the gesture you observed.*

3. Level of Emotion

Emotion words are a very common way for humans to express their experience, and will come up here and there throughout the case; but *when the focus of the conversation is on the emotions, we say we are at the level of Emotion.*

Emotions as a bridge to Delusion and Sensation: Emotions should be treated as a bridge level—it is not necessary to spend a long amount of time here unless you feel the patient is stuck at the Name or Fact level.

The level of Emotion is helpful to explore with patients who tend to stay rigidly at Fact level without much energy. For them, the level of Emotion acts as a bridge to the level of Delusion and Kingdom/Sensation. Many other people will skip across this bridge easily as one explores the level of Fact, and it is not necessary to bring them here directly by asking about emotions. There are situations where the patient is sharing a painful experience for the first time, and then it may be your role to be the listener for them, which is fine. Then, when they are done, you can move to the level of Delusion or Kingdom/Sensation based on the Vital Expression.

At the level of Emotion, you are exploring the patient's feelings. The patient will talk about sadness, anger, irritation, fear, tension, worry, joy, happiness, and so forth, which are associated with the Chief Complaint. If the feelings don't hold much energy, examine the situations or worst times in which these emotions arose. As you are listening to the patient talk about emotions, listen for Universal Language, listen for images the patient uses to explain the emotions ("it's as if…"), and watch for gestures. Once the emotion is experienced strongly, start asking them to focus on the experience of the emotion rather than the emotion itself.

If the patient mentions some situation spontaneously, ask about the experience of the situation, not about the emotions or factual details in that situation.

Level of Emotion as a Way to Confirm the Vital Expression

If a patient uses the same sensation words or Universal Language to describe an emotional state that he already used to describe a physical state, then you probably have found a piece of the Vital Expression. Have the patient expand on it briefly, and then follow immediately by dissociating him from his physical and emotional complaints. For example, a man said his cough is "violent and aggressive" and makes him frustrated. You ask him to describe the experience of his frustration, and he says, "At work I have this same frustration when my boss keeps me late—I want to attack him and cut him up, stab him!." The Vital Expression in this example is violent, aggressive, attack, cut and stab.

Spontaneous Denials Should Be Explored—"I'm not angry."

If a person strongly and spontaneously denies an emotion, that usually indicates that emotion holds some important clues to the case. Ask the client to describe the feeling further, even if she continues to deny it. For example, a person says, "Ghosts do not scare me." The question would be "Tell me about ghosts not scaring you." Then you should continue to probe into the issue with ghosts, keeping in mind that there is most likely a fear of ghosts, which the patient is denying. Or if the person says "I'm not angry at him" simply say, "Tell me about not being angry at him."

Avoiding Stories—Don't Ask "Why."

At the level of Emotion, it is not important to know *why* the patient is angry or *what* they are angry about. You, as the homeopath, need to understand the experience of his anger, the complete phenomenon of his anger, which arises from delusion, sensation, and energy. The exploration of all the levels will reveal the complete truth.

Questions to ask at the level of Emotion:

- How do you feel about having this illness?

- Describe the Experience of (angry, sad etc.)?

- Tell me more about hating (or not hating) your husband?

Questions to ask to move beyond the level of Emotion:

- What is it like for you when you feel (angry, sad, depressed etc.)?

- How do you feel in your body when you are angry?

- What is the sensation of being angry?

Bypasses: A Last Resort

Compensation can fixate patients at specific levels, where the casetaking can get bogged down. If the case is truly stuck, one way to move to deeper levels is to use bypasses. When a person cannot get past the level of Emotion and you have explored all avenues of open-ended questioning, consider using a bypass to get to a deeper level. But be careful: in adults, bypasses often lead to the wrong remedy, especially if you have not identified the Vital Expression!

In a bypass, you are asking the patient directly for an image to work with. These images have not arisen spontaneously, so they generally don't follow the natural energy of the case. Therefore, they should only be used as a last resort at this point in the casetaking. (Later on, once the patient has had a chance to explore the Vital Expression, these same questions can provide very relevant information.)

The themes that are used for bypasses are:
- Interests
- Fears
- Fascinations
- Childhood
- Stressful incidents (particularly those that led up to their symptoms)
- Favorite books, movies
- Dreams (you should always ask about dreams if they don't arise spontaneously; however, unless you need a bypass, you should save asking about dreams till the end of the case, as confirmation.)

If these areas do not elicit unique perceptions from the patient, then you can explore the patient's personality, aims, relationships, work, fantasies or religion. You can also ask them to make a doodle or drawing; then have them look at the doodle and describe the experience of looking at it. Doodles and drawings can be a particularly effective way into the Vital Expression with children. And in general, children tend to be more tuned in to their own energy (and less interested in an adult's line of questioning), so using a bypass with them tends to be more reliable.

4. Level of Delusion

Images, metaphors, dreams, scenarios: Delusion is the level where it is possible to see how the emotions are perceived and how the patient views her situation. Look for the metaphors, dreams, visual images and past or imaginary scenarios that the patient spontaneously brings up. At this level the patient commonly uses the words "it is like…" or "it is as if…" *When the focus of the conversation is mostly on these images and dreams, we say we are at the level of Delusion.*

Avoid Getting Caught in an Image

What you want to understand is not the image itself, but what is the sensory and energetic experience of the image for the patient. What was the experience in the dream? How did you experience that thing that happened in the past?

At the level of Delusion, there may be some commonly-used metaphors, like "I feel shattered," or "I felt stabbed in the back." This may or may not be indicative of the Kingdom or Kingdom information. If you think this could be the Vital Expression, simply ask the patient to tell you more about feeling shattered and stabbed, and see what comes; otherwise, just ask them to tell you more.

Image Is Not Source

The most common mistake among homeopaths using the Sensation Method is mistaking images used by the patient (to describe the "as-if-ness" of their experience) for the Source itself. Many cases use the image of a volcano to describe the experience of their pain or anger, but not until the case is explored through the levels and from the Vital Expression can we be sure the patient needs Hekla Lava. Similarly, many people use the image of being in a shell to describe alienation, depression, etc., but they don't all need shell remedies.

If you ask about the Vital Expression again and the patient uses a different image, you know it was just an image, metaphor or delusion (rather than Source language that relates directly to the remedy needed) because many different images will suffice to describe the Vital Expression.

If your question is "Tell me more about something holding you down?" and they say "It's like a tiger on my chest, pressing."

So you say "Good, tell me more about holding down and pressing.

And they say "It's like someone put a rock on my chest. I can't move it."

Do they need tiger or rock? Neither. You are not at the Energy level where the qualities of the Source are revealed.

Caution: If You Ask Them to Describe the Qualities of the Image, They Will

If someone says "it bursts out and overflows, like a volcano" and you ask them to tell you more about volcanoes, they will give you a full description of a volcano, with all the qualities. What you need to ask is more about bursting out and overflowing, not about volcanoes.

A Few Words About Dreams

If the patient does not spontaneously bring up a dream during the course of the casetaking, the practitioner should ask about dreams as part of the process of confirming the prescription. Patients' dreams always need to be explored in casetaking, and are not always on the level of Delusion. What are the significant dreams now and in the past during childhood? Do you have any recurrent dreams? What is the main action in the dream? What is the feeling of the dream? What is the sensation in the dream?

Do not ignore or interpret dreams, but trace the experiences in the dreams and get the exact description of all the elements in the dreams if it seems relevant—especially if the dream appears to contradict the conclusion you have already come to in the case. For example, you think you have a Mineral case, but the dreams are all about being chased and eaten by tigers. Ultimately, when followed to Sensation level, his dreams may still confirm the case, but check carefully before leaving a dream that contradicts your understanding of the case.

At the Level of Delusion, explore:

- Anything the patient compares his local sensation or experience to

- Metaphors and imagery the patient brings up spontaneously

- Dreams the patient refers to spontaneously

- Drawings (especially in the case of children)

- Past or imagined scenarios that remind the patient of their current situation. "It's like this time that…" (but beware of getting caught in too much story)

- Gestures, especially repeated or intense ones

To move to the level of Kingdom/Sensation ask:

- What were the sensations in that circumstance (or dream) you referred to?

- Describe your experience more—not the complaints, just the sensations.

- Describe this gesture you are making

- What do you experience in your body, when you talk about this?

5. Level of Kingdom/Sensation

Universal Language: Eventually you need to bring the patient into the level of Kingdom/Sensation, where they are focused on the description of active (rather than qualitative) Universal or non-human specific expressions ("pressure, clawing, loose, cracking, bursting, kill," etc.).

When the focus of the conversation is mostly on active Universal Language in the form of sensations and non-human specific verbs, we say we are at the level of Kingdom/Sensation. At this point the homeopath has already become aware of what the patient's Vital Expression is (and has seen how it is common to the mind and body) and now needs to understand how this Vital Expression manifests in the patient's Universal Language.

The patient sometimes enters this level spontaneously. At other times, the homeopath hears these words as they occur during the questioning at other levels and starts repeating them back to the patient and asking for more information—purposefully focusing the patient on this level, especially once the Vital Expression is identified.

At This Level You Are Building Your Direct Understanding of the Remedy

The goal here is to understand several things: the Kingdom, the Sub-kingdom, and the miasm. So if the Vital Expression is "held down and attacked," then you show the gesture, repeat "held down and attacked" with the same tone, cadence and intensity as the patient, and ask them to tell you more.

If the patient says "It's like I am fighting for my life against something bigger than me. It's a matter of survival," then you have the Kingdom—animal. So you say, "Good, tell me about held down, attacked, fighting for your life, something bigger." The patient says, "I have no way to defend myself, they have all the power, I just want to get away." Then you have a hint that maybe this is not a predator animal. You continue to feed back the words, until you have built your understanding of the remedy. If the patient names an animal, it may or may not be the animal they need. Go back to the Universal Language and just ask for more and more until the patient has built a complete picture for you of how it is.

Interplay Between Kingdom/Sensation and Delusion

When you are solidly in the level of Kingdom, you will still get quite a few images from the patient. These images tend to be more reliably related to the Source, but they are still not necessarily the Source itself. They are often markers for the Kingdom and Sub-kingdom. For example, if, in the example above, the person says, "It's like I'm a deer being eaten by a wolf," that would help to confirm that this is in the Animal Kingdom—probably a prey animal, and maybe a mammal— but not necessarily the specific animal they say. To understand the Source, you must understand what the sensation is of being attacked and held down that leads the patient to think of a deer being eaten by a wolf. They might answer "I just want to crawl back into my shell and hide."

Ask About Verbs Not Adjectives

At this level, you are still looking for Sensations and the actions that go with them to confirm the Kingdom and Sub-kingdom. Therefore, keep asking about things such as attacked, held down, squeezed, etc. but note any quality words (adjectives) that come along with those verbs (hairy, grey, heavy), since they may relate directly to the source and will help to confirm it.

Common questions at the level of Kingdom/Sensation are:

- Tell me more about (repeat back words of the Vital Expression and Universal Language in the same manner as the patient, and show them the gesture they used).

- Tell me more about (repeat words of Vital Expression) and this (Kingdom words).

- Describe more what you are showing with your hands.

- Define "x" or what do you mean by "x."

- Can you draw me a picture?

Look for the Process and Information, Not for the Name of the Source

Keep seeking and confirming the Vital Expression until it is consistent at this level. Remember it is not one thing you are observing. It can be a whole process being described.

Don't Go Backwards

If the patient goes back to facts or emotions, bring her gently back to the point and ask about the Universal language. If the patient goes back to their Chief Complaint, that is a good confirmation that the conversation still is relevant, but don't linger there because you want to keep them dissociated from their own body and daily experience in order to get them to the Energy level. Ask more about the Vital Expression and repeat back to the patient the Kingdom, Sub-kingdom and Source language that follows.

However, If You Don't Have the Vital Expression, Go Back to Square One

Some patients jump quickly into the level of Kingdom/Sensation within the first few minutes of the casetaking. If the homeopath is not aware of the Vital Expression yet, exploring the level of Kingdom will not lead to an accurate prescription. If you find yourself here prematurely, go back to exploring the Chief Complaint, local sensations, emotions, and related images until you find the Vital Expression.

Questions to ask to move to the next level:

- You have said it is "opening and blooming" and "growing and expanding" (list all the Kingdom/Sensation words they have used). What are the qualities of this "opening and blooming?" Describe it in more detail…

- Close your eyes and tell me what you experience. Any qualities come to mind—colors, sounds, texture, shapes…?

- Can you draw this "opening and blooming and growing" for me?

- Describe it in a way that I can experience it, too.

6. Level of Energy

Qualities and Patterns of Energy

Gestures, vocalizations and words that indicate the qualities of direction, shape, movement, pace, color, odor, and sound represent the Energy level. When the focus of the conversation is mostly on these qualities, we say we are at the level of Energy or Source.

Ask at the Right Time

If you observe the patient's movements (especially hand gestures), her speech (the sound, frequency, and speed), and the energy of what she is describing, you will notice patterns. Energetic qualities are present through the whole interview, but the homeopath should only focus on these qualities after the Vital Expression, Kingdom, and Sub-kingdom have been determined. The qualities you are seeking to understand are those relating directly to the Vital Expression as it is manifested in the Kingdom level.

The questions you formulate at this level need to encourage the patient to describe more about the actual qualities of the energy and gestures being explored.

Mirror Back the Patient's Energy

The more you follow the patient's energy and direct it back to them with your posture, tone, voice and gestures, the more easily they will tune into it and be able to describe it.

The energy level is mysterious to patients, and they usually cannot access the name of the Source. The energy level is far away from the region of names. It is an entirely different way of viewing the world, and most people will comment "I don't have any idea of what I'm talking about here." At that point you should say, "That's okay, I understand where we are, just keep going. This is very helpful."

Caution: Describing something already named is NOT Source language. For example, if the patient says, "it's like a horse running in a field," and you say "tell me about a horse," you will probably get a lot of relevant information about horses but this does not mean you are at the Energy level, nor are these qualities of the Source. The qualities of a remedy must be extracted from the Sensations,, not from direct questions about a substance already named. (We know we keep saying this, but it's worth repeating.)

7. Level of Potentiality

The seventh level is about potentiality, synchronicity, evolution, NOW. It is the space within which the pattern is revealed and the healing begins. It is associated with potentiality because it is simply being with the patient and watching what unfolds, leaving your head and heart open to the possibilities. When the practitioner is comfortable with this level, anything is possible.

The homeopath has to be at the 7th level, or level of Potentiality to effect change! Homeopathy cures at the level of Potentiality.

Don't give all the attention to the form—focus on the potential of the experience. It takes inner practice, like meditation, and self awareness, but you know you are there when you are listening, observing, and not thinking. The Energy in the room shifts, the clues appear, the light bulb blows in your office, alarms go off, a flock of rare birds swirls outside the window—or, as you listen to the patient, you find yourself experiencing a strange sensation. This is the formless world peaking into form—the Quantum or the gap, where deep healing occurs and evolutionary change become possible.

The delusion is still our story, in archetypal form. The strange, rare and peculiar symptoms are the clues we follow. And the Vital Expression is the doorway to go to the level of Kingdom and Energy where the Source lies. We are given the chance to bridge the worlds between human suffering and the substances that heal them through the universal consciousness, some higher power.

In homeopathy, we use words to translate the unspeakable energy patterns that influence our lives, pattern-matching to find a bridge, and remedies to stimulate a healing process. It is the Vital Force that Hahnemann describes in the Organon that brings the healing, and when the person speaks the qualities of the remedy they need, they are tapping into universal consciousness, also called the Akashic Records. It is the miracle of deep healing that we witness when a patient is prescribed a Source Remedy.

Open your attention to what is possible and just be with the patient…

LEVELS IN POTENCIES AND FOLLOW UPS

Potency

The potencies are determined by understanding the level at which the patient generally experiences their Chief Complaint and life. What level does the person naturally speak from with ease, without asking them to stick to a particular subject? Do they come in using words like "I'm so angry at my body?" Do they use image after image to describe each symptom? Do they name off every doctor they have seen and what diagnosis they gave? These are good indicators of what potency they need. If there has been a lot of suppressive therapy used, you may want to start at one level below the level at which the patient expresses himself, which may help to avoid aggravations.

The levels also tend to be correlated with where the disturbance appears to have lodged—if it is mainly a physical complaint, with no emotions associated with it, a 6c or 30c may be sufficient. In a case of depression with very few physical symptoms, a 200c may be appropriate. If a person is experiencing hallucinations or nightmares as a main complaint, consider a 1M, associated with level 4 or Delusion.

Levels & Potencies

Level 1—Name	6c	LM 1, 2
Level 2—Fact	30c	LM 3, 4
Level 3—Emotion	200c	LM 5, 6
Level 4—Delusion	1 M	LM 7, 8
Level 5—Sensation	10M	LM 9, 10
Level 6—Energy	50M	LM 11, 12
Level 7—Potentiality	CM	LM 13, 14

Follow-ups

The levels and potencies represent the patient's usual level of consciousness and awareness, as well as the current level of the disease process. So, as the case progresses and the person evolves and becomes more conscious in their daily life, they will generally need higher potencies. On occasion, as the patient progresses in their healing, they may need to move down to a lower potency. Although moving down in potency is not common, it seems that sometimes something was left uncompleted, and the recurrent emotional or physical complaint needs the lower potency in order to resolve it fully.

Potencies can be determined by the patient's level of expression in the follow ups, which can change as time goes on. For example, the patient may need a lower potency because in her general expression she went from the level of Delusion to the level of Emotion.

Many homeopaths practicing with the Sensation Method are finding that case management is very dynamic, and that aggravations, recurrence of old symptoms, and discharging are happening with more intensity and quicker. The repetition of the remedy may be helpful if the case becomes stuck or the patient wants to "do" something to move through these experiences easily. Certified Inner Health Homeopaths are finding that the repetition of the remedy in water (put 2-3 pellets of the prescribed c potency in a half liter of water, shake 10 times and then take a teaspoon) can support the patient through these difficulties. Of course, Sac-lac may also be helpful for patients wanting something to take.

It is important to explain to patients the process of aggravations and return of old symptoms. During a healthy aggravation, patients tend to move through the difficulty with a new awareness, watching it without the usual reactivity. There is a sense of ease and okay-ness about it, even though the symptom has flared up.

If there is a feeling of "stuckness" with the aggravation, it may be that the potency was too high, or that the remedy is simply incorrect. The homeopath needs to assess if the state is the same and at what level the patient is currently experiencing her Chief Complaint.

PART 6: DIFFERENTIATING KINGDOMS AND SUB-KINGDOMS

Why is Kingdom so Important?

In the past, a homeopath could be looking at remedies from multiple Kingdoms for one prescription. Even when using the Sensation Method, if you only look at the energy pattern, you could mistake one remedy for another by misidentifying the Kingdom. For example, the energy pattern that includes "floating upwards" vs. "held down" could express a plant such as cannabis, an animal such as a mammal, or a mineral such as a gas. Without clear Kingdom language, the pattern is often randomly assigned by the homeopath to the remedy with which he or she is most familiar.

The approach we outline here shows that when you reach the level of Kingdom in the casetaking, the patient will speak in more Universal Language, so that the Kingdom, the Sub-kingdom and sometimes the Source of the remedy will be confirmed. If you do not know how to tell that you are at the level of Kingdom, you may miss the information, or identify the wrong Kingdom even if the patient gives it to you clearly.

How close is close enough?

Do we have to find the "one" substance that the patient names or describes?

It seems from experience that "good enough" works in many cases. So you can prescribe Lachesis in many cases for someone who needs a snake remedy, but at some point in the case management, you may need to refine the prescription and give one that is closer to the species the patient needs.

Certain cases do require an exactness, which may mean you have to find the substance and make it into a remedy. This may have to do with the Vital Force of the patient, and the more compromised they are, the more exact you may need to be with your prescriptions.

The Different Qualities of the Kingdoms

How is the main complaint experienced by the patient?

Each Kingdom has its own distinctive nature. In basic terms, patients who need a Plant remedy will experience their main complaint as a problem of sensitivity and reactivity, patients who need Mineral remedies will experience it as a problem with structure and function, and patients who need animal remedies will experience it as an issue of victimization or struggle for survival. In addition to the Plant, Mineral and Animal Kingdoms, there are Nosodes (bacteria and viruses), Sarcodes, Fungi and Imponderables to consider. The basic Kingdom expressions will often start showing themselves early on in the case; however, it is important to confirm the Kingdom only at the Kingdom level from the language and gestures of the Vital Expression.

PLANT KINGDOM

Themes

Sensitivity
Reactivity
Adaptability
Growth
Stimuli
Polarities of sensation such as "loose vs. tight"
Shock
Absorb and release (photosynthesis, oxygen, water etc.)

Sensitivity and Reactivity

A plant is sensitive to changes in the external environment (such as weather, heat, etc.) and also capable of adapting/reacting to these changes in order to grow and thrive.

People needing Plant remedies often view their illness as an issue of oversensitivity, and can be oversensitive to many foods, medicines, and physical and mental stimuli.

Repetition and Polarity

The patient who needs a Plant remedy will often express the sensations in a simple manner, repeating the same expression over and over, or using similar expressions to say the same thing. Many times the opposite will spontaneously come out as a way to explain the sensation, such as "blocked means not flowing."

The patient who needs a Plant remedy can express this sensitivity, adaptability, and reactivity in a variety of different ways, yet it is all essentially the same phenomenon. For example the patient might say "tight, constricted, tied up" and "loose, unbound, free." These are various ways of describing the two polarities of a single phenomenon.

People needing Plant remedies are also more likely than those from other Kingdoms to have a Vital Expression that includes the same sensations as their local sensations.

As the patient moves to the level of Energy where Source language is revealed, do not be confused if the patient drops the Sensation language and starts describing a process. For example, the client says it is "pushing out (of the earth), absorbing (air), opening (to the sun)." Again, you need to know where you are in the case so that you have determined the Kingdom before understanding the Source language.

Miasms

In order to find the specific remedy from a Plant family, it is important to find the Vital Expression—whether it is reactive, passive, compensated or a more general expression, and then to perceive the miasm—the depth and intensity of how the patient copes with the Vital Expression in the different areas of their life.

Plant Sub-kingdom Information

Dr. Rajan Sankaran's "Insight into Plants" (Volumes 1, 2 and 3) and "Sankaran's Schema" have started to chart the Plant Kingdom into various Plant families and their related sensations. Versions of this information are also available in the computer programs Vital Quest, Reference Works, and RADAR.

There are many Plant remedies (including common ones) and whole Plant families that have not been charted by sensation or miasm. It is always a good idea to repertorize your Plant cases and see what else comes up that is not on the chart. Even if you are looking at a remedy that has been charted, check the Materia Medica and be sure that it fits with your understanding of the case.

If you find a Plant case with a polarity of sensations that do not match "Sankaran's Schema," you should ask the patient to describe the sensations in as much detail as possible. You can ask them to draw, or even name, the plant. If it is a known Plant remedy in the Materia Medica, you can try to confirm it with their symptoms. If it is not, and you are sure the patient was at the level of Energy, then go ahead and have the remedy made. You will be surprised how well it can work when you have followed this casetaking process.

Sometimes a patient's description will be too general, like "a large tree." If you trust their description, you will have to use traditional repertorization, looking only at tree remedies,. In the follow up or in a recase, you will be able to refine the prescription if needed.

The charting of Plant Sub-kingdoms has been somewhat disorganized, due to the enormous number of families and sub-families in the Plant Kingdom, and the various methods of organizing them. Errors exist in some of our commonly used charts.

This information is further complicated by the fact that botanists have several methods of charting relationships between plants—some based on DNA, some based more on similarities of the plants' physical and chemical properties. It is unclear which of these will prove to be most useful to homeopaths. The homeopathic programs Encyclopedia Homeopathica and RADAR allow you to look at Plant families with any of the three major botanical systems of classification, with a high degree of accuracy.

Tricky Plants

The carnivorous plants, including Drosera, will have animal characteristics, such as the feeling of being trapped, suffocated, tricked, etc. These remedies are potentized using both the plant material *and* the carcasses of the insects inside the plants.

ANIMAL KINGDOM

Themes

Issues of survival or threat to the patient's life
Victim and aggressor—me vs. you
Hierarchy
Sexuality and attractiveness
Competition
Dominance
Split within one self
Need to belong to a group

Survival

Animals rely on a huge variety of patterns to ensure their survival. But the essential problem for all animals is how to survive. For many, this is an issue of being predator or prey, for others an issue of serving a master, for still others an issue of hiding within a shell. If you think you have an Animal case, try to understand what the reaction is when threatened.

Victimization

People needing Animal remedies will often experience their symptoms as if something else is *doing* it to them. This can be experienced as a duality within themselves—such as a good side and bad side that are at war, or as if there is something living inside them that is torturing them or trying to kill them. Issues of victimization can also be experienced mainly through projection—the person may feel they are the victims of their doctors, or someone close to them, and blame all their symptoms on the other person.

These reactions do not automatically confirm Animal Kingdom—again listen to the Universal Language from the Vital Expression and see if the patient is describing the experience of an animal. It is usually a complex process, not just one or two aspects being described. For example, a tiger will have qualities of the hunter as well as the consciousness of the prey. It is important to match the energy pattern to what you see and hear.

Cycles

Animals have a complex life cycle, often with different stages. Animal cases tend to have multiple Vital Expressions that may be cyclical.

Classes and Subclasses

The Animal Kingdom is further divided into classes and sub-classes (which represent the different types of survival modes).

- Mollusks
- Arachnida
- Insects
- Vertebrates or Fishes
- Reptiles
- Birds
- Mammals

Within these, one must also distinguish between domestic and non-domestic animals, predator and prey animals, carnivores and herbivores, etc.

Differentiating Animal Sub-kingdoms and Species

Some points that help in the process of differentiation of the Sub-kingdom or specific animal:

- **Survival mode.** Do they hide and run away? Do they dominate? Do they find a place within a group? Do they kill? Entrap?

- **Type of attack.** The victim-aggressor relationship and type of attack feeling can tell a lot about which Sub-kingdom you are looking at. Does it entail speed like a cheetah? Surprise like a snake? Trickery like a spider? Is it squeezing and suffocating? Ripping and tearing? Plunging and grabbing like a bird of prey? Is it poisonous like a snake or insect?

- **Type of death.** Sudden death is often found in the insect world, where they can be stepped on or swatted at. Life seems easily and quickly threatened. In herd animals, death is more often the result of straying too far from the group or becoming weak and not able to keep up. Some animals, such as lions, will fight to the death with another lion, and therefore death can be the result of competition and hierarchy.

- **Hiding and Camouflage.** Some animals rely heavily on masking themselves and only give warning when the threat is very close. For example, the snake remedies often have the issue of deceit, and can use this skill when being interviewed so that they can look very mineral-like until they are gingerly coaxed out of hiding or suddenly feel threatened (at which point you will have no trouble discerning which Kingdom you are in!).

- **Pace of the energy.** The energy patterns of smaller animals, spiders, and insects generally move faster than larger ones.

- **Group dynamics.** In herd, pack, and flock animals, there are issues of belonging vs. not belonging, taking care of members of a group, and levels of hierarchy and leadership.

- **Diet.** Are the animals herbivores or carnivores? Pollen gatherers? Water filterers? Sometimes people will make reference to the food source of the Animal remedy they need. One woman needing Apis had repetitive dreams of fields of flowers.

- **Miasms.** Snakes tend to be Syphilitic, as do lions. Most other mammals (lac remedies) tend to be Sycotic. Insects and birds tend to be Tubercular. However, a specific remedy prescribed at Source level could be any miasm.

Hard to Spot Animals

Some sea animals can be harder to spot than other animals. For example, the sea anemone, which is plant-like, will be very sensitive and not easily express animal characteristics. Shelled sea animals, including corals and sponges, may use Mineral type language, and the victim-aggressor characteristics will be downplayed.

In animal cases, it is often necessary to rely on your casetaking skills at the level of Energy to find the exact species that the patient needs. The Animal remedies, especially bird remedies, are very under-represented in the repertory and material medica and are not easily charted. So, when you know you need a bird remedy, your only recourse is for your patient to give you all the details, so you know you need, for example, sparrow instead of canary at the level of Energy.

Animal Sub-kingdom Information

Our Animal Kingdom remedies as a whole are not well-proven. Our classical Materia Medicas have far fewer Animal remedies than plants, and modern provings, which are heavily weighted towards mental and emotional symptoms, don't usually bring out as much pathology as would be helpful.

This is somewhat balanced by the fact that most people have much more general knowledge of the life cycle and behavior patterns of animals than they do of plants or minerals. However, this knowledge must be used with caution.

We have a lot of ideas about animals, and what their experience must be like, but if we use this sort of information, we are often wrong. Universal Language that occurs in the Vital Expression approach to casetaking will not always fit your idea of what snake cases are like, or what sea remedies should sound like. It also may have nothing to do with your ideas about what that animal's life might entail. Nancy Herrick's proving of Lac Equinum, for example, brought out a degree of suffering that most horse owners would be shocked to read about, even though they think they understand horses. And bird cases could express their whole state from the perspective of being in a shell.

Be careful if an animal is mentioned in the case, check for what does not fit in the patient's description. You must seek to understand the qualities being expressed without getting stuck on the animal stated in the case.

There are numerous reference books on animals that are helpful to differentiate specific remedies. These include Dr. Jonathan Shore's "Birds: Homeopathic Remedies from the Avian Realm," Massimo Mangialavori's "Bitten in the Soul: Experiences with Spider Remedies in Homeopathic Medicine" and Nancy Herrick's "Animal Mind, Human Voices: Provings of Eight New Animal Remedies," as well as "Sankaran's Schema" and the software program, "Vital Quest."

Natural history reference books, and internet research is often helpful and necessary for differentiating Animal remedies. The more you learn about the behaviors of different animals, the better equipped you will be to distinguish them when they wander into your office and start describing or acting out these behaviors with you.

MINERAL KINGDOM

Mineral Themes

Structure
Function
Organization/disorganization
Performance/role
Development
Relationships
Work/Task
Completeness/incompleteness
Building/Lack/Loss of capacity or energy
Void—matter vs. non-matter

Creation and destruction of matter

Structure, Capacity, and Function

Minerals bond and break down in differing arrangements in order to create and destroy the structures of the universe. They perform functional roles in their differing states of matter. The flow of the periodic table charts the development from energy, to matter, to dissolution of matter.

Something is Missing

People needing Mineral remedies tend to see their illness as a problem within themselves, something wrong with them, an essential void or something missing, a lack of development of capacity, or a loss of capacity. They may describe this problem as a process that is not going properly—a bump in the road, a slowing down, a narrowing, a collapse of a structure, etc.

What is Missing?

In looking for Sub-kingdom and Source information (column, row, and specific remedy), you need to determine first what is the essential nature of what is missing or not happening (which row), and is it something that still needs to develop, or something the person has already fully developed but then lost (which column, left to right)?

Minerals and Levels

Confirm the rows and columns only after you have confirmed the Vital Expression and are hearing Kingdom language. At the Fact and Emotional levels, most people needing Mineral remedies will talk about problems with work or relationships—but they are not all needing fourth and third row remedies. (Be aware that many people who do not need a Mineral remedy at all can describe their symptom as inhibiting their ability to function.)

Mineral Source Language Isn't Always Helpful

Once the Kingdom and Sub-kingdom have been confirmed, one often needs to drop back down to the Delusion level to understand the exact remedy needed. There are times when the Source language will help to differentiate two similar Mineral remedies. However, Source language in Mineral cases isn't always that useful, so don't spend too much time there unless you are already quite clear where you are in the periodic table.

Salts and Compounds

In a Mineral case, the patient can need an element alone, or in combination with some other element, as in a salt, a compound, or a particular mineral-based substance such as Hecla lava. Ask yourself the following:

Does one element alone explain the Vital Expression of the patient completely?

Does the patient express the theme of more than one element in their Vital Expression and at the level of Delusion? Is there an essential conflict between two or more themes? The Vital Expression is a wonderful tool in salt or compound cases, because when you probe one aspect of it in depth, the patient will want to remind you that you are missing an element or elements, and this will help you to understand how to find the salt or compound.

In Carbon cases, where the remedy is often a compound with Hydrogen, Nitrogen or Oxygen, you will hear themes and Source language from these individual elements, along with the general carbon issues. The discovery continues as we uncover the Carbon world, thanks to Dr. Roger Morrison's work in his latest book on the Carbons.

Progress in our Understanding of Minerals

The current process of differentiating Mineral remedies is to understand the Vital Expression, confirm the Mineral Kingdom at the level of Kingdom, and then go back to Delusion level and even Fact level (which is often Delusional in Mineral cases) to understand the themes and images that are currently associated with the rows and columns. This method, which relies heavily on Dr. Jan Scholten's work, has already given us a huge breakthrough in our understanding of Mineral remedies and their relationships to each other. However, we are poised and ready for the next step, which is beginning to happen.

With the recent work of several homeopaths, we find there may be concepts and Universal Language that identify the rows beyond the common method of understanding the delusion or situation in the case.

Dr. Andreas Holling, in his chart, *Dimensions of the Periodic System,* shows how energetic language and gesture may relate to different rows.

Dr. Jayesh Shah has proposed that "grip," "falling", and "pulling down" sensations could be a theme for all of column 3, which we previously only recognized in Borax.

Spero Latchis is exploring the idea that oscillating or changing references in the Universal Language could indicate an odd numbered stage, and more stable or fixed Universal Language could be an even number stage.

These theories are all cutting edge, and will need to be confirmed as we gather and analyze more cured cases. But if these ideas prove to be true, they will help enormously to eliminate the confusion that can occur when one differentiates Mineral cases only by themes and delusions related to rows and columns.

Periodic Table Reference Materials:

Jan Scholten contributed an enormous amount to our understanding of Mineral remedies by his analysis of the Periodic Table of the Elements according to homeopathic thinking. His books and charts are useful as references.

Dr. Andreas Holling has introduced a theory of the level of Kingdom language and gestures for the rows.

Jayesh Shah's book, *Into the Periodic Table*, is helpful in understanding the gradual development and loss of structure as the columns go from left to right.

Dr. Rajan Sankaran's *Vital Quest* software program is a useful resource with its added information about the periodic table, as is *Sankaran's Schema* with its charts.

Dr. Roger Morrison's book *CARBON Organic and Hydrocarbon Remedies in Homeopathy* is useful for identifying a Carbon remedy.

NOSODES: BACTERIA AND VIRUSES

The Nosode expresses a mode of defense against a particular infection or disease which becomes generalized. Since miasms are reflections of a disease state, in a Nosode case, you will hear the coping mechanism of the miasm expressed in every sphere of the patient's life, though it may not correspond to the miasms with which we are already familiar.

There have been so few Nosode cases taken in the Sensation Method that we are just beginning to understand what they might sound like from the patient's language. Frans Vermeulen and Jenni Tree's work in the book, *Monera*, has opened doors to understanding Nosodes from the perspective of bacteria. Jenni Tree's lectures on Monera show themes to aid in recognizing a possible Bacteria Kingdom case.

Jenni Tree summarizes the Monera Kingdom below:

> In the case taking, we may be confused by the fact that the patients seem stuck on the fact level. They talk of nothing but disease in some way. The miasm seems to be very strongly represented. This is because the miasm is the disease. The Vital Expression is Source language, yet we are confused because it seems like Fact level.
>
> I think a Vital Expression for a Nosode must have to do with movement, evolution, going somewhere, changing—it has to do with motion. Bacteria are in constant

motion. This explains why Rhus tox and Pyrogen are so often well-used in acute inflammatory conditions. However, our intention in using the Sensation Method is to treat chronic levels as well, so we must listen for the voice of the Monera Kingdom— the voice of the bacteria and virus.

BACTERIAL QUALITIES/ IDEAS / THEMES

- *Contagion, Communication, Colonization, Commensalism*
- Altruism –working for the common good
- Helpful, symbiotic, co-operative, social, democratic
- Opportunism
- Creative, strategists, evolutionary, genetically flexible
- In a patient needing a Bacterial remedy, we will see a history of fevers, inflammatory disease, childhood illnesses, digestive upsets, catarrh, and muscular rheumatic pain.

Like humans, bacteria are worse for overcrowding, poor nutrition, unsuitable atmospheric conditions of temperature, oxygen, and pH; and Interference. Left to their own devices, they will find a balance in their situation. Interference in that balance, whether through pharmaceutical drugs (e.g. antibiotics), surgery, change in diet, invasion of other bacteria, or any change that the Vital Force cannot withstand, will create action on the part of the bacteria. It is possible that, at this point, the peacefully co-existing bacteria become Pathogenic.

Some bacteria—anthrax and clostridia botulinum, for example—are naturally highly toxic. The work they do produces toxins, which most humans have insufficient vitality to overcome.

PATHOGEN QUALITIES/ IDEAS / THEMES

- Toxicity
- Speed, Quick reacting, Fast evolution
- Migration
- Aggression

Pathogens are the most 'acute', fast, voracious and vicious members of their group. Like the alkaloids in plants, they are pure vital substance. A little of a pathogen goes a long way. They are evolved and adapted for maximum efficiency.

VIRAL QUALITIES /IDEAS / THEMES

- Desire to influence, Control, take over.
- Infection
- Intimacy
- Force
- Hiding
- Change, mutation
- Information

And What is the Sensation of this Monera Kingdom?

- There is something about **movement**, motion. This connects with the bacterial need for **evolution**.

- Evolution is a need for **change**. We can see the **hectic** state of tuberculosis here.

- Possibly because of this need for movement, there is something about **speed**, **hurry**, or **slowness**, the sensation of everything moving very slowly around one, or of things being speeded up, whizzing, **vibrating** like a standing motor.

- When we think of life being speeded up to a pitch that we cannot imagine, then we get jumps in time, and a confusion of the sense of **time and place.**

- Perhaps we have a sense of being lost in well-known places, or of well-known places looking different, or we get a sense of **déjà vû**, or of repeating actions we have done earlier.

- **Imitation** comes to mind. Syphilis – the great mimic – whose place is rapidly being taken by Borrelia burgdorferi, aka Lyme disease. **Things are not as they seem.**

It is difficult to find the information. All the old nosode cases were taken on the fact level. Nosodes were used as a "never been well since," an intercurrent remedy, or to move on a blocked case, etc. We have very little sensation or Source language as yet. The above language and sensations are taken from Medorrhinum, Streptococcus, Brucella, Tuberculosis, Borrelia and Typhus cases.

FUNGI

Sankaran's Schema still places fungi on the Plant chart, yet in nature they stand in a Kingdom entirely their own, with a subdivision for the Lichens. From what we know at this point, Vital Expression, when explored in the Fungi Kingdom, is expressed as spreading, invading, and taking over. Many fungi in our Materia Medica are drug remedies.

Jenni Tree, Editor of *"Spectrum Materia Medica, Volume 2, Fungi,"* summarizes the Fungi Kingdom:

The role of the Fungi on the planet is one of *transformation*. There are other ideas which support this:
- Reduction - from complex to simple;
- Recycling, Decomposing, Replenishing;
- Maintaining an intimate relationship with the environment.

The Fungi are as necessary to the Plant Kingdom as the Bacteria are to the Animal Kingdom.

Some Fungi themes, Sensations, ideas from a recent Psilocybe proving are:

- Infiltration, invasion
- Manipulation, Deceit
- Trance, Doors of perception
- Rebellion, violence, increased strength
- Wholeness, togetherness, fragmentation
- Enlargement, expansion, vortex, contraction, being inside oneself and unreachable
- Tightness, bandaged, stiff, carapace, trapped, restricted, squeezed in versus expansion, held wide apart
- The space between things expanded, visible
- Dream, deception, madness, things not as they seem
- Vertigo--moving up
- Vortex--the still point of the moving world
- Time being out of joint or distorted
- Water

Fungi Themes from Frans Vermeulen's *Spectrum Materia Medica, Volume 2, Fungi*

- Transformation
- Penetration
- Extension
- Expansion, Branching
- Pioneering, Colonising
- Absorption
- Adaptability, Flexibility, Resilience
- Invisibility -the Fifth Column - Renegades
- Specialists
- Strength and Survival
- Decomposition
- Speed, rapidity
- Energetic, active
- Cheerful
- Alcohol
- Cold - low body temperature
- Desire carbs, starch, nitrogen, processed foods, liquids
- Better or worse in dry and humid conditions

Fungi share characteristics with the Insects, so be aware of this when choosing the Kingdom. They share chitin, (the tough semitransparent substance that forms insect wing cases and fungi cell walls), restlessness and activity; energy, strength and survival; the ability to penetrate (or sting as with insects) and the desire for liquid or processed foods.

SARCODES

Sarcodes express the healthy function of one part of the organism (hormones, for example), which becomes the main issue for the entire organism. The indication for these remedies will be very clear Source Language at the Level of Kingdom and Energy.

IMPONDERABLES

Imponderables are expressions of qualities beyond matter, space and time. Some examples are Magnetic poli ambo, Microwave, Electricitas, Cell phone, Sol, etc. The confirmation of these remedies in the case must be at the Energy level where the Source language is clearly articulated.

PART 7: MIASMS

What are Miasms?

Miasms are dynamic energy forces that inform the organism of the pace, mode, and depth of its own destruction and recovery process.

Miasms lay down the patterns of susceptibility of a particular individual, and the paths through which an individual will attract and contract certain maladies. The miasm mandates the pace at which an illness will progress and the modalities it will express. Along with each miasm come tendencies towards certain emotional and personality traits, as well as certain delusions and behaviors.

Miasms affect groups as well as individuals

Miasms also affect social groups, such as families or entire societies. We frequently find families manifesting one specific miasm in different ways, or find children in a family expressing the predominant miasm of either the father or the mother.

A Brief History of Miasms

Hahnemann himself wrote of his discovery of miasms:

> This invaluable discovery, of which the worth to mankind exceeds all
> else that has ever been discovered by me, and without which all
> existent Homeopathy remains defective or imperfect...

Yet Hering disagreed:

> What influence can it have whether a physician adopts or rejects the
> Psoric theory so long as he searches for the most similar medicine
> possible?

One of the practical problems inherent in Hahnemann's legacy of miasms is that he left no comprehensive description of any of the miasms, or any type of map that would allow his followers to easily explore his enormous discovery. Instead, he listed numerous symptoms of Psora and elaborated long lists of remedies belonging mostly to the Psoric miasm, and shorter lists for Sycotic and Syphilitic miasms.

Kent concluded that the theory of miasms did not belong solely to the medical sphere: "It goes to the very primitive wrong of the human race, the very first sickness of the human race, that is, the spiritual sickness."

Ortega ascribed very specific characteristics to each miasm: he said the main idea of Psora was inhibition, for Sycosis it was excess and for Syphilis, destruction.

George Vithoulkas brought up the miasmatic theory in more recent history, and was likely the first one to propose that homeopaths don't need to feel limited to three miasms, but that it was possible to consider that Tuberculosis could be another miasm in its own right.

Miasms raise the question of the meaning of health and disease, which can be looked upon in life as a process of evolution. The challenges of a disease can support a significant growth in the person. Many patients who had cancer attest that they feel they grew a lot or are better people after facing cancer. The same is often said by people who are recovered alcoholics.

This concept resonated completely with Hahnemann's own very revolutionary concept of health for his time. Health is what the human being needs "so that our indwelling, reason-gifted mind can freely employ this living, healthy instrument for the higher purposes of our existence."

Harry van der Zee, in *Miasms in Labor*, challenges the traditional negative concepts of disease and miasms: "Miasms offer us the struggle that helps us connect with our invincibility, the darkness that makes us discover the light in our soul, the destruction that makes us aware of the indestructibility of our eternal being."

How can these concepts help us as homeopaths in our daily practices? For one thing, they remind us that the ultimate aim of homeopathy as a medical science is not to just treat disease, but to help human beings in their evolutionary path.

Sankaran's Classification and Use of Miasms

In the 1990s, Sankaran created a classification and definition of specific miasms (including several in addition to the ones identified by Hahnemann) that can be recognized in the patient and confirmed through the Vital Expression. In Sankaran's view, the miasm can be seen as a coping mechanism and can be identified by the depth and degree of desperation in the patient.

Sankaran also showed that in a case the patient perceives only one miasm, usually beginning at childhood, and which does not change with circumstances.

Listening for the Miasm

The Vital Expression and the miasm are two aspects of the same experience, which the patient experiences as a single phenomenon—his disease state. Therefore if you ask about the sensation, the miasm can be elicited: "How do you experience this tied up feeling?" "It makes me feel hopeless." Likewise, you ask about the miasm, often the Vital Expression will be elicited. For example, you might ask, "What is it that you experience so hopelessly?" and the patient replies "I feel hopelessly tied up." This hopelessness could indicate the Syphilitic or Leprosy miasm.

- **Just listen.** In order to determine the miasm, often times there is no need to ask a direct question; instead, listen to the way the patient presents his main complaint and how he is coping with it.

Questions the homeopath can ask the patient in order to find the miasm

- What is the effect of the Chief Complaint on you?

- How do you perceive your Chief Complaint or situation?

- How do you react to and deal with your Chief Complaint or situation?

- How hopeful or desperate do you feel in this situation?

Cautions about Miasms

- **Pathology does not equal miasm.** The pathology is only a partial expression of the disease state and does not necessarily determine the miasm. Therefore, not everyone with cancer needs a Cancer miasm remedy, and not everyone with skin problems needs a Ringworm miasm.

- **Miasms are not to be determined by single words.** Be aware that the use of certain key words by the patient does not necessarily indicate the miasm. For example, if a patient uses the word "control," it does not mean the patient is in the Cancer miasm.

- **Miasms are a continuum, not a static point.** A remedy may have qualities of the miasm indicated before and after it.

Interactions between Kingdom and Miasm

Miasms in Mineral Cases

The Vital Expression of a Mineral case will be expressed around issues of structure and function, which will be more Universal Language (i.e., pressure, heavy, balanced, etc.). The miasm is how the patient views and experiences his issues of structure. As a general rule, the periodic table tends to go from Acute to Syphilitic miasms as it progresses from top to bottom. However, this is only a broad overview, and cannot be applied rigidly. Each remedy needs to be viewed independently for its miasmatic characteristics. For example, Alumina is in the second row and often is found to be a Syphilitic remedy. However, Hydrogen is in the Acute miasm.

Miasms in Plant Cases

Plant families contain many members, which are being classified into various miasms. If one looks at a chart of Plant families—such as in *Sankaran's Schema*—one or more plants from the family fit in each miasm. Our understanding of Plant families and miasms is still evolving, and the chart is therefore incomplete and should be seen as provisional.

Miasms in Animal Cases

Remedies from each Animal Sub-kingdom often share the same miasm. For example, insect remedies are often Tubercular miasm, but not necessarily. Many mammals are Sycotic miasm, and many snakes can be Syphilitic. Again, each remedy needs to be understood individually.

Miasms Can Help Determine the Sub-kingdom

In Animal and Mineral cases, the miasm can sometimes be helpful in determining the Sub-kingdom when the Source is not completely clear.

The understanding of miasm helps in differentiating between remedies that may have similar symptoms. For example, Sulphur and Platina share the symptom egotism. The Sulphur ego is optimistic and not very desperate (Psoric). The Platina ego is very desperate and can lead to suicide or homicide, and feels altogether quite hopeless (Syphilitic).

How to Differentiate the Miasm from the Vital Expression

It can be difficult to differentiate the miasm from the Vital Expression, especially in Plant cases. The miasm is more the way the person copes with the illness, the sensation is more how they experience the illness. The forced out sensation of the Liliiflorae family could be confused with the cast out theme of the Leprosy miasm. If it is Leprosy miasm, there will also be feelings of disgust, dirtiness, etc.

Let's take an example: The patient has the sensation of being suffocated. Is this the Vital Expression of the Rosaceae family, or a remedy such as oxygen, or a constricting snake, or is it the Tubercular miasm? If it is the Tubercular miasm, there should be other aspects of the miasm present, such as feeling hurried. If suffocated is the sensation and not the miasm, it will not have the other miasmatic indicators present.

If the patient says that they feel suffocated and hurried, and they need to escape in all areas of their life, then the homeopath has to ask how they feel suffocated. The patient may answer that it feels like cutting, stabbing, pinching, etc., in which case it could be a Tubercular remedy of the Ranunculaceae family.

As the case progresses, the differentiation should become clearer. Be careful not to make quick assumptions—bearing in mind that the miasm and the Vital Expression are often tied together in Plant cases, and can be confused.

Many times, as the Kingdom language is revealed from the Vital Expression, the miasmic expressions will come spontaneously. In some cases you can ask specifically: "How do you experience this sensation?" and then the patient will explain the miasm to you. In other cases, you will review all the clues given in the case, keeping in mind that there may be language of other miasms, especially the ones before and after.

Ten Miasms — Ten Ways of Coping

Acute — Panic
Typhoid — Crisis
Psora — Struggle/Hopeful
Malaria — Hindered
Ringworm — Trying
Sycotic — Stuck/Avoiding
Cancer — Control
Tubercular — Trapped
Leprosy — Cast out
Syphilitic — Destroyed

Acute Miasm (Panic)

In the Acute miasm, the situation is perceived as temporary but life threatening, as in an acute disease—an intense threat of massive proportions, a sudden, great danger to life that pops up without warning. The attitude is one of sudden panic—a jump, a shriek, a shock, a freeze, an instinctive fight or flight response such as you would feel at the very moment you rounded a corner and came upon a tiger, or upon suddenly feeling an explosion right outside your door. In the Acute miasm, the patient is only focused on the panic and does not focus on how to resolve it, and because they are only in that moment, there is no sense of hopelessness, even though the situation may in fact be dire.

Typhoid Miasm (Crisis)

The patient feels himself to be in an urgent, life-threatening situation requiring his full capacity to get through it, as if he was a parent watching a building on fire with his child inside. The situation is perceived as being so urgent that the patient is willing to use any means to return to a secure position—violence, scheming, lying, etc.

The feeling is, "If I can just get through this crisis, I have it made and I can rest." He is rushing around and seeking help. In the Typhoid miasm, the patient is primarily focused with all his intentions on how to get this situation resolved as quickly as possible. This is why the Typhoid patient will call you at any hour to get your help, whereas the Acute patient is in such shock it will not occur to them to get help.

Psora Miasm (Struggle/Hopeful)

The feeling is of a difficult situation (but not a crisis) where one has to struggle in order to succeed, like a student studying for final exams. There is anxiety with doubts about his ability, but he is hopeful, and failure does not mean the end of the world. He must struggle in order to recover or maintain his position.

Malaria Miasm (Hindered)

The Malaria miasm lies between the Acute and the Sycotic miasms. The person perceives an acute threat coming up intermittently in a situation that cannot be changed because of a fixed feeling of deficiency. This is like a woman living in an abusive situation, where she feels stuck with the knowledge that, at unpredictable times, she will be attacked for no apparent reason, yet she feels incapable of getting herself out of the relationship.

Ringworm Miasm (Trying)

The situation of the Ringworm miasm seems to be one at the borderline of the person's capacity. There is hope of possible success with a cheerful quality, and so there is a lot of effort, but each failure makes him give up and accept his limitations. This is more like someone trying to learn something he is not very good at—such as someone with dyslexia trying to learn to use a computer. It is not a crucial task, but he really would like to know how to do it, so he keeps trying. The classic example of Ringworm Miasm is a person trying to lose weight, who gets all excited at the beginning and then fails, and then is resigned to being overweight, until they get excited again.

Sycotic Miasm (Stuck/Avoiding)

The Sycotic attitude is one of acceptance, avoidance, hiding and cover up of the situation they cannot deal with. Such an attitude comes after a long unsuccessful struggle with the problem. The problem feels stuck and constant, so it is best to avoid the situation. This situation can be compared to an adult who has never learned to read but who doesn't want anyone to know, so he avoids situations where his secret might be found out.

Cancer Miasm (Control)

The Cancer miasm lies between the fixity of the Sycotic miasm and the destruction of the Syphilitic miasm. The sensation is perceived as chaos which is going out of control leading into destruction. The person feels he has limited abilities to bring the situation back under control, but he is the only one who can do it. The person is trying with all his might to keep control in a situation that is really desperate, such as a pilot trying to sound calm and collected while knowing that the flight is probably going to crash—trying to fly the plane while everyone else is panicking.

Tubercular Miasm (Trapped)

The Tubercular miasm lies between Sycotic and Syphilitic, where the situation is viewed as desperate and oppressive, like being stuck in a mine shaft with very little air, or chased down an alleyway by someone much larger than you. There is a sense of time ticking away, and a need to escape. The patient may appear burnt out from the hectic pace. There is very little hope, and destruction seems imminent.

Leprosy Miasm (Cast out)

The Leprosy miasm is close to the Syphilitic miasm, with similar destruction, desperation and hopelessness. What is different is that in the Leprosy miasm, there is a tremendous feeling of rejection, dirtiness, and self-loathing. The attitude in response is violent, despair, and almost beaten. The patient's focus is on their disability or inability to succeed. There is this sensation of being so hopeless that nobody would want them. The only glimmer of hope is that they may succeed after all, with nobody's help, and thus humiliate those who shunned them. In our society, this might be compared to a person who is constantly rejected and humiliated by their classmates because of a severe disfigurement, and has fantasies of revenge.

Syphilitic Miasm (Destruction)

The experience of the sensation here is very deep, so much so that it seems permanent, destructive and fatal. This compels an attitude of complete hopelessness and either intense desperation or extreme despair. With the Syphilitic patient you must be concerned about their literal survival. There is a real possibility of suicide (or homicide) with these patients, so if you have a Syphilitic case and they are talking about suicide, you must take them literally and act accordingly. There can be a chilling seriousness and calmness about their attitude, since they feel there is nothing left to do and no hope. This can be compared to the attitude of the sniper, who kills without feeling, and then one day decides to kill himself, since he feels life has no meaning whatsoever.

The Value of Miasms

Miasms are not always as helpful as we had originally hoped in the selection of the remedy. However, recognizing the miasm in a patient's case will help you with prognosis, case management and overall understanding of the health of your patient. If we all take careful note of our patients' miasms and keep track of how they respond to treatment, we will learn more about the role of miasms and how they work, and develop better tools to manage our cases.

PART 8: THE FOLLOW-UP

Casetaking is only the first step to choosing a remedy that will act deeply, resolve the Chief Complaint, work even during an acute, and support the patient in an overall sense of well being. The next step is to analyze the case and make a prescription. But the tough part comes later, in the follow-ups, when we see how the remedy does over time.

I just saw a great case of....

Many people excitedly report that they have a great case of such and such, and when you ask them how long it has been, they say they just took the case last week, but they are SURE that they know the remedy. We all do this, and it's fun to share the excitement of a new case. The danger is in thinking you have learned something about a remedy when the results of the case are still unknown.

Homeopathy Works

Luckily for all of us, homeopathy can work very well even when prescribed on keynotes or delusions. However, those cases typically do well for a time, and then need recases after several months, or even after a year or two. It may be that the remedy was close enough, and then needed further refinement, or that the energy pattern was very similar, even though the Kingdom was not the same in the recase when using the Sensation Method. It does appear that there are analogs between Kingdoms. More clinical case reviews based on the Sensation Method will help us to know for sure if there are analogues between remedies taken at the Kingdom level or not.

Pile-ups of Poor Prescriptions

Unfortunately, during the months where a relatively unknown remedy prescribed on a delusion *is* working well, we can delude ourselves as practitioners that we now know everything about this remedy, and prescribe it in other cases that are even further off course from the original wrong prescription. At the end of the year, you may have four "cases of Positronium," none of which are working. This sort of thing can be a hazard to your practice, not to mention your patients themselves.

Aggravations

The concept of aggravations can aggravate the situation, as many poorly trained practitioners insist a remedy must be working as the patient is getting worse and worse. We must keep a careful eye on our egos when we are so sure of our case analysis skills that we forget to care whether our patients' symptoms are actually improving. Aggravations, if they occur at all, should be brief, and the patient should have a sense of "okay-ness" at their center, an inherent sense that things are improving, even though certain things may feel worse.

If you have recurrent problems with aggravations, then start patients at one potency lower than the one indicated. Of course, the use of LMs can also support a more gentle process in some cases.

So what are the clues that the remedy is working?

Improvement of Symptoms

Obviously, we want to see the symptoms improve. If the patient is not feeling better after a few weeks, then either the prescription was wrong, or the potency was too low (nothing happened) or too high (severe aggravation). Some cases have severe pathology, and will take time to see significant improvements. Do not change remedies if the patient is moving in the right direction; only consider changing if there is absolutely no change after you have tried different potencies. Do not change remedies during an acute, because this is an ideal time to check your prescription. Repeat the constitutional remedy and consider going higher in potency if needed. Don't doubt your prescriptions until you have seen how they work. Have your cases reviewed by someone knowledgeable in the Sensation Method before changing your prescriptions too soon.

Volume Gets Turned Down

The recovery of our patients can also be seen in the "turning down of the volume" of their Vital Expression. When the Vital Expression is probed in a follow up, the gestures and expression should be quieter, less extreme. After six months of successful treatment, you should take a more in-depth follow up to see if this is true. This also may be true of the miasm.

It Works in Acutes

Most practitioners of the Sensation Method find that in Source-level cases, the remedy works in acutes. It is not necessary to do a full retake if you are quite sure of the remedy. However, acutes are a great time to check and explore the Vital Expression if you have any doubts about your choice of remedy. The Vital Force tends to speak loudly and clearly during acutes, and you may find yourself able to confirm Kingdom, Sub-kingdom and Source very quickly.

What Difference Has it Made for You?

When Jayesh Shah hears that a person's symptoms have improved, he always asks the question, "And what difference has it made for you?" The answers to this question could be a textbook of good health. People report feeling a sense of freedom far beyond the simple lack of a symptom. Something is lifted, a door opens, and things fall into place that they never thought possible.

Synchronicities

When a remedy truly fits the patient's energy pattern, synchronicities can occur, which indicates a deeper level of healing is occurring. A man, still living with his mother, who was the source of many of his problems, reports that his mother has suddenly decided to move to her own place. Health is the ability to be in the flow, attract positive energy, dispel negative energies, live in harmony and resolve challenges in a profound way. This sort of health is possible through homeopathy.

Does the lion in the human disappear? Or just become a healthier lion?

This is the Zen koan of the Sensation Method. Everyone sees it a little differently. Rajan Sankaran states unequivocally that a cured case of Lac leoninum is not a healthier lion or a better behaved lion, it is simply a human being. Others feel that you can never totally remove the tendency towards the vital disturbance, and that the best that can be hoped for is an extremely well-behaved lion that you could invite to dinner at your grandmother's house. Is there a difference? We're not sure.

Are there different layers of remedies?

This is another unresolved question in the Sensation Method. Many homeopaths agree that *in general* there is usually only one remedy state that goes back to childhood. Dr. Jayesh Shah says he has seen cases where there were two remedy states in one person, and the person would alternate states every now and then. Both remedies worked, only one was needed at a time, but as one state cleared, the other would sometimes appear. This question will be answered through clear documentation of all our clinical cases over long periods of time using the Sensation Method to have any degree of accuracy.

CONCLUSION: THE IMPORTANCE OF COMMUNITY

Ask for Help

In some cases, you will not be clear of the Kingdom, Sub-kingdom or the specifics of the remedy based on the Source language. At this time, the collaboration of homeopaths who are using the Sensation Method can be helpful. First, your colleagues can check whether the case is well taken and the information is clearly stated by the patient, or if the case is simply not clear, and you need to go back and get more information. Then there are homeopaths who are more familiar with certain Sub-kingdoms and can help to make sense of what you are seeing. It may be a very well-taken case, and you are simply unfamiliar with the remedy. Sometimes we are looking too closely and thinking too much, and another pair of eyes can see it more clearly.

Working in Community

Wherever you live and work, you should try to find some way to share successful cases with your colleagues and get supervision with difficult cases. This is important even for those of us who have been doing this work for many years. The Sensation Method of casetaking was *not* the development of one brilliant homeopath working in isolation. These ideas developed through meetings of a group of homeopaths in Mumbai, India ("the Bombay Group") all sharing their knowledge, experience, and observations. The Sensation Method has continued to be refined by the additional observations of homeopaths around the world.

Start a study group in your area, attend workshops, and share your cured cases.

Inner Health Subscription Service. Inner Health offers *Homeopathic Services*, a monthly subscription service to support colleague-to-colleague help. Many of these issues of case management, potency selection, and differentiation of Sub-kingdoms are also being researched and discussed through the Homeopathic Services bulletin board and monthly teleconferences.

New Clinical Materia Medica Studies. Inner Health is also publishing a new series of clinical Materia Medica Studies on particular Sub-kingdoms, and is looking for input from others using these methods. If you would like to participate in any of these projects, contact Alyson@innerhealth.us. Or visit www.infohomeopathy.com to sign up for the Living Homeopathy eZine to keep up to date with new information and services that may help you with your cases.

Clinical Bird Cases. Inner Health is also currently seeking clinical bird cases for common extractions of symptoms. Please email your bird cases to alyson@innerhealth.us if you have at least six months of good follow ups.

An Evolving Materia Medica

As homeopaths, our successful cases will become the future clinical Materia Medica necessary for its refinement. The ongoing process of extracting rubrics and language of cured cases at various levels will help us differentiate remedies within a Sub-kingdom much more precisely in the future. Your careful work at this stage will be an aid not only to your own clients, but to many generations of homeopaths—and their clients—in the future.

We each play a role in the future of this work. Please join us in this endeavor.

APPENDIX:

**Hypothesis about the DIMENSIONS OF THE PERIODIC SYSTEM
for Homeopathic Materia Medica, according to A. Holling**

E	R	Space Dimension	Physical Dimension	Sensation	Variation	Left & Right Side	Gestures	Themes
H, He	1	Non-localization 0 dimension	Field, non-localization	Matrix background, canvas, no differences. Ouroborus, non-existence, pre-existence, source of being.	No			Feeling as if not noticed, not to exist; delusion has no bones.
Li - F	2	Existence Localization Manifestation Place / subject 1 dimensional	Place, location, point, origin, separation from the source of being, the undifferentiated – existence by separation (the relation is not important).	Subject Existence Separation from the source of everything Birth	The degree of separation from the source, birth	Left: Existence as separation hardly realized. Right: Expansion of existence; loss of existence, existence is threatened by death; separation more than necessary.	Nitricum: The expansion of the localization. Showing boundaries with hands.	Separation, birth, the structure of independent existence develops.
Na - Cl	3	Relationship Connection Translocation Translation Object and way, distance 2-dimensional	Distance between two points that are related to each other; linear, motion from A to B, direction, the horizontal dimension. The plane– two points–distances longer and lesser, linearity. Two things: one or the other.	Objects Two entities, two locations, direction, difference, identification, clearness, definition, discrimination.	Motion Distance Direction Discrimination	Left: objects direct subjects. Right: subjects direct objects. The object at the mercy of the subject.	Two-dimensional hand gestures, horizontal motions, vectors, arrows, linearity.	Identity, choice, decision. Reach the destination, reach, arrive, distance.
K - Br	4	Accumulation Storage Transport Reality Space energy-storage 3-dimensional	Work = force x distance [Joule] Energy is stored work, the charge, weight, motion against resistance – with effort – volume, room. The force is proportional to mass $(E = mc^2)$	Power, energy storage, the charge, potential force. The new dimension is the force: lifting, pushing, carrying, transport, invest energy, fill.	Charge, amount of energy stored, weight and mass	Left: A structure needs more force to move. Being charged, being filled. Right: A structure needs to regain the force necessary to overcome an obstacle.	Hand gestures indicating space structures: cubes, balls, hills, mountains.	The secure space/room; the house: you have to defend against danger (have to invest power into the motion). [Normal] work expectations, guidelines, inputs, benchmark and fulfill the role, to fill out; to overcome, surmount.
Rb - I	5	Event Episode Transformation Reality Time 4-dimensional	Performance = work/time [Watt] Space-Time. To manage space-time, you need information (messages). Information will be stored instead of energy, to anticipate changes in time. Transformation	Time, to predict the future, forecast; to have time issues, e.g., deadlines, timeframes, etc.	Information Knowledge Prediction Illustration of the change of form	Left: To need information, not knowing timely changes. Right: to know everything; to not forget; too much information, filled, stuffed. Transcend by knowledge.	Time is difficult to illustrate by hand gestures.	Skill, special ability, special performance, presenters, singers, musicians, sports people, aggravated by a deadline. If a time is set: guides, advice. Storage of knowledge, e.g., DVDs, books, etc.
Cs - At	6	Causality Determination to govern, to rule Cause Responsibility Effect 5-dimensional	Effects: A cause affects events.	Intention, effect, cause, determine, initiate, force, rule	Effect	Left: Cause and determination are others – this structure is not developed. Right: Causality should exist, but is difficult to establish.	Effects are difficult to show by gestures.	Responsibility, power, leadership, desire for causality, religiousness.

About Melissa Burch, CCH, RsHom(NA)

Melissa Burch, CCH, RsHom(NA) co-founded The Catalyst School of Homeopathy with Christopher Beaver, CCH. She established live phone case supervision and clinics based on the Sensation Method. She created a unique homeopathic phone referral service with a homeopath team approach. She is president of Inner Health, inc., which produces numerous online and onsite courses for homeopaths, homeopathic patients and people interested in alternative medicine. Her advocacy for homeopathy in the U.S. is ongoing, including hosting a 12 hour video marathon on UStream for World Homeopathy Awareness Week, and produced the first Radio Series on Homeopathy. She was the Master Homeopath for the proving of Stoichactis Kenti Sea Anemone. She co-wrote and published the four part manual "Dr. Rajan Sankaran's Correspondence Course," and "Vital Expression: A Manual on Homeopathic Casetaking." Ms. Burch worked with Dr. Nandita Shah at Quiet Healing Center in South India for over a year and half. She graduated from the School of Homeopathy New York, directed by Jo Daly, and the New York School of Homeopathy, directed by Robert Stewart.

ABOUT INNER HEALTH, INC.

Inner Health (IH) provides homeopathic services to the general public and to the homeopathic community. IH is a leader in establishing the highest quality of services in the complementary and alternative medical field through its education, practitioners, workshops and services.

IH's vision is to make homeopathy a household word. Our goal is to identify IH in the consumer's mind as the place to go for the best, natural deep healing on all level—mental, emotional, physical and spiritual; and to create a demand for homeopathy and in particular for Certified IH Homeopaths, through our innovative, educational and creative marketing materials.

Training

IH provides basic and post-graduate training for homeopaths to develop reliable and better results in their practices by following the IH Approach—a systematic way of case taking and analysis based on the Sensation Method—and by implementing the IH System, which includes case management protocols, scripts and information, client business services and marketing.

Homeopaths have the opportunity to train and become Certified IH Homeopaths through workshops, supervision and educational materials. Combined with our own extensive marketing of IH and the IH approach to homeopathy, which results in constant referrals to Certified IH Homeopaths, IH Homeopaths will have a unique and wonderful opportunity to develop themselves as professional homeopaths, heal others, share clinical information with the homeopathic community, be well paid and have excellent systems to guide them to provide the highest care to the client.

www.ingramcontent.com/pod-product-compliance
Lightning Source LLC
Chambersburg PA
CBHW080054280326
41934CB00014B/3309

ISBN 9780989342902